What Do We Eat Tonight?

How to Live with Food Allergies

by Dianna Barra

A Practical Guide to Selecting Foods and Creating a Rotation Diet.

Included are a variety of charts to help you get started on a rotation diet and to help you successfully stay on a diet plan.

Written in short chapters, this book is designed to help you get started with as little effort as possible to adjusting your diet and getting on the road to better health and most importantly, still enjoy life.

Tested over 15 years, these methods and hints have helped improve not only the author's health, but also the health of her family, friends and many others.

The information in this book is for the purpose of education and information only. This Book is not intended to diagnose or prescribe for any illness or give medical advice. It is not to replace the care or advice of a licensed healthcare professional.

Content

Published by:
Idea Designs: Instructional Designs for Every Application, LLC
5515 North 7th Street, 5-285
Phoenix, Arizona 85014-2531

orders@idea-designs-online.com
http://www.idea-designs-online.com

ISBN, Print Edition. 0-9711370-0-5
ISBN, PDF Edition. 0-9711370-1-3

First Printing 1998
Second Printing 2002, completely revised

Printed in the United Satates of America

Cover, Illustrations & Design - Michael Swaine Design and Illustration

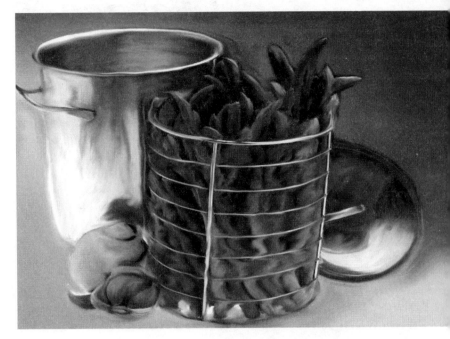

Acknowledgements

Many thanks to the following for their support and contribution to this project.

Joanna Lewis, Dr. Robert D. Milne, Chris Zgurich, and The Morgan Family to get me started on this project.

Michael Swaine, Graphic Design; Patricia Johnson, editor; Susan Ward, typist who helped immensely with production.

Without their help, patience and encouragement it would never have gotten finished.

Lastly and most importantly to my mother Maggie Barra, who put up with this project for the last few years.

4

Preface

This little adventure started when several of my friends started to inquire about my healthy eating habits. I decided that it would be handy to put the information into book form so they could refer back to it when needed instead of just hearing about it once.

If you can't tell, eating healthy food is one of my soap box items that I feel really strongly about. But, because of my introverted personality, I would rather write about it and if someone is interested in reading it, that is fine, rather than joining a national organization and going on a public crusade for better food. I will editorialize on a few items in this book, but I think that you can easily tell what is my editorializing and what are the facts that I have observed.

The information in this book is a compilation of over 15 years of being on a very strict allergy diet, advice from my doctor, advice from my dietician, my experimentation, my background as a chemist, working in a pharmacy, and the many books that I have read.

As one person noted, it is easier to tell what is wrong with a person than to cure them. If you choose to follow some of the suggestions that I have learned from these sources over the years, remember a couple of things. First, you get as much reward out of something as you put into it. So, if you follow the suggestions to the letter, you will get more benefit from them than if you cheat. Second, be aware of your current medical needs. Don't compromise any existing situation. Check with your physician before any change. But, the bottom line is...who ever DIDN'T benefit from eating better and more nutritious food? I hope that you enjoy this book and that it is helpful to you!

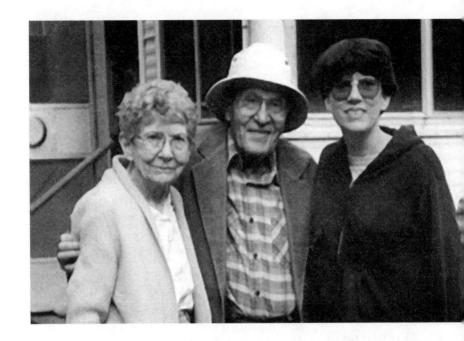

Our Story
Our Quest for Better Health

My mother has always fed us very well and in a "health food manner" even before it became "fashionable". In the early 1960's I remember going to "health food stores" and "juice bars" and eating "good" vegetables. I have always tended to be a natural foods eater and an environmentalist. (Who else would try to recycle plastics as early as 1973?)

Later in life, I kept eating healthy food. But as time and the pressures of school became greater, I started to not eat as healthy as I should have. (Besides, those jelly-filled doughnuts looked REALLY good, and EVERYONE knows milk is good for you!) When I started getting really sick, I reverted back to better and healthier food and I began to feel better. However, this was not enough. After suffering for ten years with feeling bad and getting worse and having friends and doctors saying "You're just getting old" (at 30?), I finally found a doctor that knew what was wrong.

A major part of the problem was food and food source (food additives) type allergies. By changing to a whole food and food allergy-type diet, I am a lot healthier and more energetic than I have been for 13 to 14 years. (I also lost 20 pounds of food allergy fat, fat which I gained every time that I ate the trigger food. (No, one of the trigger foods wasn't fat, it was wheat and/or gluten). I would sometimes gain 5 pounds literally overnight after I ate a gluten containing food.) Every time that I would cheat or go off of the diet, I could tell sometimes within minutes.

Five years after I was properly diagnosed, Mom got really sick. The doctors said, "It could be allergies. Just take an antihistamine." For months she suffered and just got worse and worse. When I finally talked Dad into letting me take her to my doctor, she was a mess. But knowing that food allergies was a major part of her problem too, she adjusted her diet and as long as she would stay on her diet, she would be wonderful, which is great for a 90 year old. But, whenever she would stray off of her diet, she would get lost in her own kitchen and be very forgetful. Once she would get back on her diet, within a week or two at the most, she would be back to her old self......cooking, cleaning, vacuuming, paying bills, washing, etc. She has no high blood sugar, no heart disease, no arthritis, and her blood work levels are all within normal values. She recently had a very minor stroke at 89 years. All three of her sisters and her father never reached that age as they had died much earlier from stroke related conditions. At only 4 months from the stroke onset date, she was 80% recovered and the neurologist was extremely pleased with her recovery progress. She is great, especially compared to other women near her age. How many people even reach 90, let alone have her quality of life?

The final motivation for this point of view of life and eating was when my father at 87 years old was diagnosed with dementia during the summer of 1996. After asking the doctor what to do (a doctor whom Dad had chosen and said he liked and trusted because he thought Mom's and my homeopathic doctor was a quack) and the answer was basically "nothing", I started to take matters into my own hands. With my background and my experience, and Mom's experiences with food, I started to analyze Dad's behavior. I noticed that he would sometimes cough until he was choking when he ate. Sometimes his nose would start to run when he was eating. He seemed to pass out after eating at times, not knowing where he was and finally sleeping for hours. He had trouble breathing and complained constantly about it. With some vitamin advice from a registered geriatric nurse, I enlisted Mom's help and we started logging what he was eating when he had these symptoms of coughing, nose running, etc.

Within a few weeks we had it pretty well pinpointed to what foods were his trigger foods. We eliminated them, and changed some eating habits and Dad's health improved to where instead of lying in bed and complaining that he couldn't breathe or just sleeping all day, or wondering who we were or what day it was, Mom and I had a hard time keeping track of him. One minute he would be outside cutting the grape vine back. The next minute he would be out raking leaves. Then he would be planting bedding plants in the front flower garden or fertilizing his trees. For five straight years he earned "The Golden Age Gardener Award" in the State Fair while taking a prize on every one of his entries including "Best of Class" awards.

He started to learn to play the piano, work on his computer, and had just finished the seventh volume (approximately 600-pages in each volume) of a popular novel and enjoyed telling mother what had happened last. He couldn't wait until he could get volume eight! At his last doctor's visit for his regular 6-month check up, the doctor commented that he (the doctor) hoped he was in as good of health as Dad was when he was 89 yrs old. Dad had no blood sugar problems, no high blood pressure or high cholesterol, no heart disease, a normal PSA test, and no arthritis. This was the second time a physician had made this comment to Dad. Dad's health insurance even gave him a rebate because he had not had to make any claims on the insurance. The final proof that food allergies were a main part of the problem was that when Dad went off of his diet even for one or two meals, all of his symptoms would immediately start to return. When he got back on the diet, he would return to feeling better. True, it was not scientific, but it worked for me. (Dad passed away at the age of 90 years as the result of a root-canal that did not heal properly, it abscessed, the tooth pulled, and then through several errors of the Dental and Medical personnel, he lost his fight for life.)

Living with the food and environment allergies that I do, and reacting to foods and toxins like I do, and having seen how my parents reacted to foods and toxins, I have often wondered how many of our ills of cancers, auto-immune diseases, hyper-activity and rage, are caused by environmental toxins and a poor or contaminated food supply. How many times have a product or additives not been tested long enough or the researchers didn't notice an undesirable side effect? Or how many times were actual test results not released as was the case with cigarettes and their cancer link? We really don't know. But, this possibility is really brought home when more thorough research is showing more and more that environmental toxins are responsible for more and more of our sickness. (Refer to "Is This Your Child?" Doris Rapp M.D.). Consider too, the new information about aspartame, M.T.B.E., chromium, and other deforming chemicals in many water supplies. It really makes one wonder if we escaped one "Silent Spring" just to be caught in another "Silent Spring" a few years later. ("Silent Spring" by Rachel Carson, is still worth reading today and is still in print.)

I have noticed that even the pets seem to have been affected by this contamination of the food supply. My two cats, Whitey and Yellow were grossly overweight and lifeless, when I fed them as directed with popular healthy canned cat food. They tipped the scales at 25 pounds and 22 pounds respectively. (If human, they would have been close to 400 pounds, the vet told me.) I could not get their weight down by cutting down their food portions, and had no success even with special diet food from the vet. Everything that I tried for over a year failed. So, finally, I got some health food books about cat care and changed their diet to natural whole foods. They easily lost 10 pounds each and are so energetic at 12 years of age that they continually tear up the house. I had better not be in their way when they run down the hall as I might get run over. They have easily been their slimmer selves for over 6 1/2 years now. What a relief!

Further evidence for eating good, pure, whole foods is in my observation of people. I notice that the ones that eat good, pure, whole foods are within weight limits for their height, more energetic than others, and have fewer colds and flu and other illnesses. A big plus to eating better!

I know that tracing and eliminating food allergies and eating pure, whole foods have greatly helped my family. I have often heard the phrase that "Americans inhabit a country full of food and yet the people are starving to death." The more I experience, the more truth there seems to be in that statement. I hope that you will be as successful as we have been by changing your eating habits.

(NOTE: If you do not suspect food allergies, but just want to eat more healthy, still follow the general guidelines that are outlined.)

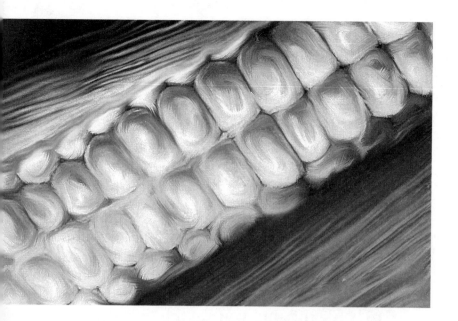

Food Allergies

If you suspect food allergies, in one way, feel relieved. Food is one of the easier things to control in the environment. It is more of a correct choice whether to eat something that you are allergic to or not, than to choose to come in contact with other allergens. Pollen allergies are controlled by the seasons and the trees, flowers, grasses, and weeds that are planted around and the times of year that they are in their pollination mode. Wind-blown allergens are sometimes hard to control. Animal dander is somewhat controllable. Chemical pollutants such as cigarette smoke, car exhaust, glues, paints, pesticides, perfumes, and potpourris are harder to avoid in places necessary to go to such as work, school, stores, airplanes, and churches. Food, at least you have some control over.

In dealing with food allergies, the most important thing to do is to listen to your body. Any hint that I give you will be of most use if you use it in addition to listening to your body. As one person said, I'm the "weapons supplier" to battle this, but you are the "general." Since you know how YOU feel, you call the shots. Since each body is different and each allergy situation is different even in the same family, listen to your body.

Some of the things to listen for are the following. Is something hard to swallow? You may be allergic to it. That was the symptom for me and my allergy to celery and oats. Are you repulsed by the smell of something? That was the way it was for me and chocolate. (Yes, chocolate!) Do you break out in a rash when you eat something? (Pork and wheat for me.) Or, do you have a craving that once you get something, you want more and more? (Milk and rice.) Do you suddenly feel tired or confused after eating something? (Dad and ice cream...sorry Dad.) These are all clues to watch for.

In the study of food allergies, what doctors call the "sinister seven" is eventually brought up. These are seven foods that a person who is allergic to food will most often react to. They are wheat, corn, milk, sugar, soy, chocolate, and yeast. The first step is to eliminate all seven of these foods and anything that contains these foods. For most of us, this will be a major adjustment. "What will I eat?" is the next question. In the following chapters I will cover the safe foods and give suggestions of how to replace these sinister seven in your diet. I know it is possible as I have done it for the last 15 years. And yes, I still have a life. It will take EFFORT and DISCIPLINE. But, try it for at least one month without cheating and see how you feel. It usually takes at least one month to clear the allergy causing foods out of your system.

Also, listen to your body. If you get any of the symptoms above (hard to swallow, craving, nausea, rash, or suddenly go tired) when you eat or drink anything, eliminate that item too. Get the combination of foods that works best for you.

One major thing that works well with food allergies is to rotate the foods that you can eat. This means that instead of, for example, having rice every day because you are not allergic to rice, you have rice one day, and a different grain the next. This will be better explained in the next sections and in the chapter titled "Rotating Your Foods."

Realize too, that some foods that you are allergic to you can still eat, but only in small quantities. This group of foods you can reintroduce into the diet on a rotation-diet basis and tolerate them with no problem. Other foods you will not be able to reintroduce into the diet ever again. Those are the facts of life...

Another thing to keep in mind when you are developing a rotation diet is that some foods go better together than others and are easier to digest when eaten together. This food combining will be woven into the discussion and be covered in the chapter titled "Food Combining."

In Summary:

1. Listen to your body.

2. Eliminate the "Sinister Seven": wheat, corn, milk, sugar, soy, chocolate, and yeast.

3. Eliminate any other food that you feel that you are sensitive to, or have been told you are sensitive to.

4. Try not to cheat for at least one month.

5. Rotate the foods you can eat.

6. Realize that some foods will be permanently out of your diet, while other foods can be reintroduced into the diet, but only on a rotation basis.

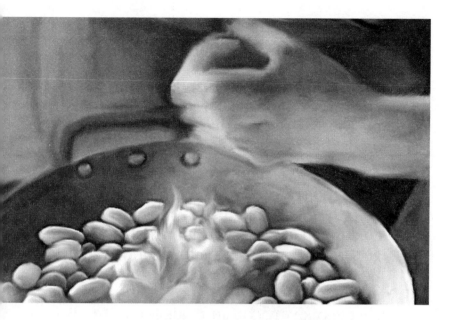

Preparing Foods

Preparing cooked foods correctly is important in any allergy or regular diet. Since we eat food to gain energy, our food needs to be prepared the best possible way to retain as much energy as possible.

First: NO MICROWAVE OVENS!!!!! It is not fully understood yet, but food contains a form of energy that when it is microwaved, it literally becomes dead food because the energy has been taken out of it. Any respectable health food person NEVER uses a microwave, not even to reheat something! (There are several studies currently going on about the effects of microwave cooking on health. The preliminary data is very much against using microwaves to obtain healthy cooked foods.) Instead of a microwave, steam, bake, sauté, fry, or roast your foods that need to be cooked.

Second: Use stainless steel or enamel pans for stove top cooking. Reports are still out, according to some, that there is no harm in cooking in aluminum. But, when aluminum gets pitted, tastes up the food, and even gets holes eaten in it by the food it covers, do you really want to take a chance? (HONEST! A cheese cake my cousin made for a party was covered with aluminum foil. When we took the foil off, it was full of holes.) One study reported on the radio which talks about alzheimer's states, "Is there a link between alzheimer's and higher than normal aluminum in the body?" They conclude that "The aluminum is a result of and not the cause of alzheimer's." With all of the news stories today of how there have been untruthful reporting in the effects of M.T.B.E., chromium, smoking and second-hand smoke on people, just to mention a few items, do you really want to take a chance? Be safe. Use stainless steel or enamel.

What about Teflon? No way. Who wants particles of Teflon in the food or bits of the plastic spatulas that are used to clean the pans in the food? Not me! Use stainless steel or enamel.

Steam vegetables in a stainless steel steamer basket. Bring the water to a boil BEFORE you put the vegetables in the steamer. This "flash steaming" locks in more of the freshness and makes nice crisp vegetables that are not over-cooked, but yet tender and done. Use water that has been purified by Reverse-Osmosis (R-O). Why go to all of the trouble of getting good vegetables and cooking them correctly, but then contaminating them with polluted steam from boiling polluted water?

For baking, use glass, enamel, or stainless steel baking dishes or roasters. Again, why go to all of the trouble of obtaining good food and then spoiling it by cooking it in the wrong pot or pan.

In Summary:

1. NO Microwave Ovens !!!!! (Not even 10 seconds to reheat !!!!!)

2. Use stainless steel or enamel pots and pans on the top of the stove. No aluminum or Teflon.

3. Use stainless steel, glass, or enamel dishes for baking.

4. Steam vegetables with a stainless steel basket steamer using only R-O water. (Remember to heat the water to boiling before adding the vegetables.)

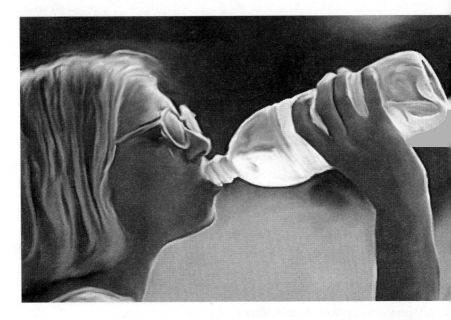

Water & Other Drinks

Water in the diet is very important. Our bodies are made up of mostly water. With all of the water ads out there, which is best?

Currently, Reverse Osmosis (R-O) purified water is the best. But as new systems are developed, it pays to keep checking for better and more efficient filters.

Spring waters may have some minerals that are not desirable depending on the spring it came from.

Some bottled waters have calcium and other

minerals put back into it to make it taste better. Other bottled water is just bottled "city water" sold at a fancy price!

City tap water can be THE WORST!! In recent years, there has been the revelation of a "plume of death" called "The Dragon" which is composed of toxic chemicals in the city water tables near Phoenix, Arizona. (See January 12, 1997 edition of the Arizona Republic newspaper.)

Just ask the person who claims he has a rare form of cancer from drinking that city tap water what he thinks of tap water. His lawsuit for damages is still in the court system. Even more recently and in the news headlines almost weekly for a while has been the revelation about the contamination of methyl-tertiary-butyl-ether (M.T.B.E.) the gasoline additive, in most of the ground water in places where M.T.B.E. is used. Being readily dissolved in water, the scope of the M.T.B.E. problem and the associated clean up has not yet been determined. The long-term health effects of M.T.B.E. are still unknown. (We are finding out that this is yet another example of a chemical hastily approved and not tested thoroughly.)

In the city of Mesa where I used to live, and Phoenix were I now live, we can get an analysis of the well or other water that we use. Having a chemist background, I was totally shocked at the chemicals in the water. Even though these chemicals are in trace amounts, "unharmful", according to E.P.A. standards, I don't want even a trace in my water! Bromobenzene, dibromomethane, and chloroform are just three of the 20 dangerous chemicals in the water.

I sure am glad that I have a R-O system to purify my water. Cost? Under-the-sink do-it-yourself models are about $200. Counter-top models are about $150. My first counter-top model lasted me 10 years with changing the filter every year ($50). Cost of water I figured to be (Yes, I taught math) about 15¢ a gallon. Lot better than hauling it from the store or paying $1.25 a gallon for someone to deliver it. A counter-top model is portable if you move and very attractive. The difference in my water bill was not noticeable.

So in choosing your water, check your source of water and filters to get the best and purest water you can.

The amount of water to drink in a day is important too. The recommended amount is 8/ 8-ounce glasses a day. I personally drink over one gallon of water a day. Yes, this means that you have to go to the bathroom more, but one of the purposes of drinking water is to help rid your body of toxins. Drink a lot. Drink at least a half-gallon a day. (That's only 8/8-ounce glasses a day. Approximately 12 swallows at a time.)

Drink water between meals, not during meals. Drinking during meals dilutes stomach acid and hinders digestion. This is important if you have trouble digesting your food.

Fruit and vegetable juices are good too. But, you have to be careful that the juice is 100% juice and not a lot of added sugars and corn syrup. Organic juice is the best to buy.

However, NO SODA POP!!!!! All soda pop is sugar water with flavoring. And definitely, NO artificial sweeteners especially NO aspartame!! Artificial sweeteners are turning out to be worse than real cane sugar, according to some studies. If you have to have something that fizzes, try some of the natural sodas. They come in many of the same flavors you are used to.

Eliminate all drinks hot or cold containing caffeine. Not only is caffeine a known stimulant of the central nervous system, heart, and respiratory system, but it can also affect blood sugar, cross the placenta in pregnant women, cause nervousness, insomnia, headaches, irregular heartbeat, panic attacks, and in some cases convulsions. In addition to all of that, in a report (Spring 1998) out of Brigham Young University Cancer Research Center, Dr. Kim O'Neill, a microbiologist, strongly suggested that caffeine may keep cancerous cells from dying when they should have died in the body. So, even though caffeine has not been proven to cause cancer, it may "encourage" cancerous cells to live longer than they should have.

Caffeine naturally occurs in coffee, cola, tea, and kola nuts. (Kola nuts are commonly in carmel, chocolate, cocoa, walnut, and root beer flavorings.)

Substitute caffeine-free grain drinks for something warm on cold mornings. Switch from cola sodas to water, fruit juices, or natural caffeine-free sodas.

For milk substitutes, there are some acceptable rice, oat, or almond-based drinks. These are good substitutes on hot or cold cereal and in other places you would use milk.

In Summary:

1. Drink pure water preferably Reverse Osmosis purified.

2. Drink at least a half-gallon a day. (8/ 8-ounce glasses)

3. Drink between meals.

4. Make sure any fruit or vegetable juices are ORGANIC and have no added sugars or corn syrup in them.

5. Drink no soda pop or related drinks with sugar or sugar substitutes. Especially no drinks with aspartame added.

6. Eliminate all drinks, hot or cold, that contain caffeine.

7. Use rice-, oat-, almond-based drinks instead of milk for cereals, and other places you usually use milk.

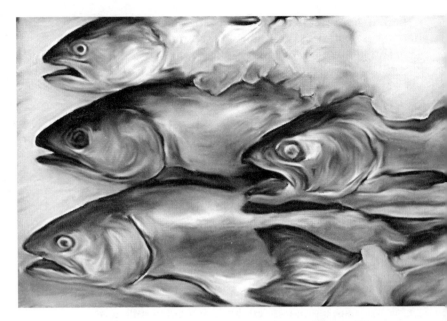

Meat
& Proteins

Meats are the basis of the American diet. Which ever ones that you are not allergic to, continue to eat them. The main key is to eat the leanest possible meats, NATURAL meats if at all possible, and rotate the meats you do eat.

Beef. Red meats are a real American staple. Since I am sensitive to all red meats, I have to be very careful when eating them. I can not cheat and eat any red meat except beef, but only if it has been rotated into the diet and only if it is hormone- and antibiotic-free.

Whatever red meat that you choose, try to find an all-natural meat with NO growth hormones or antibiotics in it. Several reports in late April 2000 strongly suggests that the antibiotics that are given food animals such as cattle and chickens may be part of the cause of the growing problem of bacteria that is resistant to all known antibiotics. Be safe, choose antibiotic-free meats. There are several brands available of hormone- and antibiotic-free beef. IT DOES MAKE A DIFFERENCE.

Our whole family can tell the difference between the natural beef and regular store beef. Cost? Very comparable in some cases, and worth every penny! When on sale, it can even be less expensive than regular store beef. Additional benefits are that it tastes LOTS better, it is usually more tender, contains less fat, freezes and thaws smoother, and contains less gristle. Once when I served some dinner guests natural beef, their child ate three slices of roast when the mother had apologized ahead of time that the child would probably eat only one-half of a slice if even that much. Even my Dad ate twice as much beef as he used to because "it tasted so good". That was important for an 89 year old.

Poultry. Choose all natural with no growth hormones, no antibiotics, and preferably "free range." (Remember "All Natural" is a Buzz word today. So buyer beware. Even arsenic is "all natural". It's an element.) Yes, natural, antibiotic-free chicken does tastes better and smoother. It is really surprising how good it tastes compared to the other conventionally raised poultry.

23

Fish. Fresh if possible. However, fish from local streams here still have D.D.T. in them which was banned over 30 years ago. A big effort has been made to clean up the pesticides and mercury in the rivers, lakes, and oceans, but much still needs to be done. Possibly the best source for good fish is farm raised fish. However, there are some experiments with genetically engineered fish to make them grow faster in fish farms. With the lack of long-term research on the fish and the people who eat these genetically engineered fish, stay away from genetically engineered fish.

Cured Lunch meats. ALL of the regular store brands are walking chemical plants with potassium nitrite and sodium nitrite added to the cured meats to enhance taste and preserve color. Many tests, some as early as 1970's, have shown that these two additives combine with natural stomach acid to create nitrosamines which are very powerful cancer-causing agents. Currently, the FDA, the USDA, and the cured-meat businesses seem to have reached a compromise on these dangerous additives while they battle safety/consumer appeal issues. Mean-while, the bottom line is that these two highly dangerous additives are still in most cured-meats and are affecting our health. Don't use them! Instead, there are some good brands of natural nitrate and nitrite-free type turkey and chicken bologna and hot dogs that are WONDERFUL. Use them instead. Be warned though, that because they are not full of chemicals, they have to be kept frozen until they are used. When using them, take off the needed frozen hot dogs and put the others back, not letting them thaw. Take off the needed slices of frozen bologna and immediately put the rest back in the freezer to preserve freshness.

To easily rotate the meats, do it alphabetically. Beef one day, chicken the next, and then fish. This gives you a three-day rotation with the meat that you fix for dinner one night is the next day's lunch. (Yes, I do pack my lunches. This is real world stuff.) Actually it makes deciding what to serve for dinner easier since I can say "It's beef night, how do I want it prepared?" That is important for a person like me who REALLY DETESTS cooking and wants to spend the least amount of time possible in the kitchen.

Meats are easier to digest with vegetables that are of the green-leafy and non-starchy variety. Usually two servings of vegetables with one serving of meat is preferred.

If you are not allergic to eggs, use them in the diet. Eggs can be served as a main dish or used in other foods. Free range and fertile eggs are better. Besides tasting better, the shells are thicker, and the yolks are less likely to break prematurely than caged and non-fertile eggs. Organic eggs are also available.

These organic eggs are produced by chickens that have been fed only organic grain.

Another source of protein is the legume family of dried beans. By combining the correct foods with the correct type of beans, complete protein meals can be achieved. A vegetarian can use this diet as a frame work for planning meals.

Other sources of proteins are nuts, avocados, cheese, and olives. However, they contain more fat than other proteins.

If you are sensitive to milk and milk products, feta cheese is sometimes tolerated as well as almond cheese and rice cheese. Be aware that soy cheeses can not be used if there is a sensitivity to soy beans.

In Summary:

1. Select all-natural meats with no growth hormones or antibiotics.

2. Choose all-natural lunch meats which contain no sulfates, nitrates, nitrites or other preservatives in them.

3. Rotate meats. (Red meat, poultry, seafood, legumes.)

4. Dried beans and other legumes are a good source of starchy proteins.

5. Nuts, avocados, cheese, and olives are sources of fat and proteins.

6. Eat any of the proteins with green-leafy, or non-starch type vegetables.

7. Almond and rice-based drinks and cheese can be used as a protein substitute.

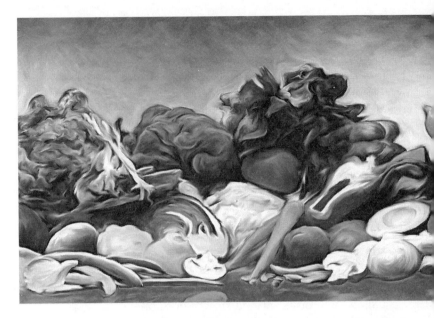

Vegetables

Vegetables are the best power foods possible. I used to laugh at vegetarians, but now, I can see the wisdom of a vegetarian-type diet. But, the vegetables need to be ORGANIC if at all possible. "You are what you eat" relates to the vegetable plant too.

If a plant is grown on chemicals and pesticides, no amount of washing will get rid of the chemicals from the inside of the plant. And with so many vegetables being grown in other countries that have no restrictions on pesticides, you never really know what may be on the vegetables either. So, try and buy organic vegetables when you can. However, the fact is that organic vegetables are not available all year, nor are they available in all cities, towns, or places. If you can't get organic, get the best quality vegetables possible. Remember, there is a growing demand for organic vegetables and more organic vegetables should soon be available for longer periods of time.

ORGANIC vegetables taste a lot better than conventionally grown vegetables. I sometimes wonder if people have to use so much seasoning on the conventionally grown vegetables to flavor them because they plain don't taste good. Well, ORGANIC tastes SO much better, that you can't believe that it is the same vegetable sometimes. Dad ate a lot more vegetables and always said they tasted great when they were organic. He barely ate vegetables when they were conventionally grown. Back to my dinner guests. The young girl even surprised her mother by eating all of her vegetables and asking for more when she was served organic vegetables. (A HAH! Is this the secret to get children to eat their vegetables????)

And talk about organic tomatoes, they really taste like tomatoes! Not those bland things that pass for tomatoes in the standard grocery stores. And the best thing about organic tomatoes is that you don't have to scrape wax off of them before you can eat them. I just hate that! Wax is basically safe. But, it can come from insects (beeswax), animals, petroleum, or plants. Some waxes have chemical additives such as pesticides or fungicides added to them to help preserve the vegetable or fruit. One can have an allergic reaction to the wax or one of its additives. Since most of the waxes on a piece of vegetable or fruit are not labeled with ingredients or source of wax, avoid waxed vegetables and fruits if at all possible.

In addition to better taste, I found that some vegetables are only edible to me if they are organic. For all of my life (40+

years), I could not tolerate carrots. They really made me gag. When I switched to ORGANIC carrots, they were sweet and edible. It was apparently just my body saying "no" to the chemicals that the non-organic carrots had in them. I have found the same experience to be true with green peas, beans, beets, and cucumbers. Now that I switched to all organic, they are edible. Even my cousin who detested carrots really liked carrot juice from organic carrots for the first time in her life.

Another advantage of buying organic is that you have less of a chance of unknowingly buying genetically engineered vegetables, fruits, and meats. With the advances of modern science, genetically engineered (G.E. or G.M.O.) vegetables, fruits, and meats are now available. They differ from other foods in the fact that the genetic structure is manipulated at the D.N.A. level. This is vastly different than the cross-pollination and selective growing and breeding that has been going on for centuries. This manipulation allows the scientist to splice the genes of different plants and sometimes even animals, or insects, and micro-organisms into a current strain of vegetable, fruit, animal, or fish. Plants and vegetables can therefore end up with genes from animals or fish in them. Certainly this is something that Mother Nature would not let happen naturally.

To create a genetical engineered plant or animal, a host micro-organism, usually a bacteria which is antibiotic resistant, is introduced into the cell of the plant or animal to be modified. The culture is then treated with antibiotics and any unsuccessful modifications are killed. The successful modifications are then grown to see which have the desired traits, the scientists killing any undesirable plant or animal if it does not die naturally.

Because of this process, scientists have made corn that gives off a scent that kills the corn worms. They have also made produce and fruit that stay fresher longer. One scientist even made a glow in the dark potato by combining a potato with the glow gene of a fire-fly. This may sound great at first, but, the corn that killed its insect pests, also killed thousands of harmless migrating butterflies that just happened to drop by. This was an unexpected side-effect. But, what other unexpected side-effects may have happened and may yet happen?

Some vegetables have peanut genes spliced into them. It improves the vegetables, but the effect on a person who is highly allergic to peanuts is still unknown. There are no labels stating that "this fruit or vegetable has been genetically altered, people with peanut sensitivity beware." Could a peanut sensitive person have a reaction by eating this peanut altered vegetable? We just don't know. Some of the most commonly genetically engineered vegetables and grains are tomatoes, yellow squash, soybeans, canola, eggplant, corn, and potatoes.

The long-term effects of these genetically engineered fruits, vegetables, and meats are still being evaluated on people, insects, and other animals. We really don't know how safe they are. However, it is a known fact that many European countries will not allow imports of genetically altered foods. Also many U.S. companies will not use genetically altered corn or other crops in their products.

It is surprising to find that currently, almost half of the U.S. corn and soy crop are planted with genetically altered seed. It is even a more alarming fact that almost all of our food supply has been contaminated by genetically engineered products. You may not realize it, but almost all of us have eaten at least several items that were genetically engineered but didn't know we were eating them. Be on the safe side as much as you can. Buy only organic and non-genetically engineered vegetables, fruits, and meats.

When planning your menu, green leafy and non-starch vegetables can be eaten with anything. With two servings of vegetables at each meal, you easily get your four servings a day.

Rotate your vegetables by family groups. For example, cabbage, cauliflower, broccoli, and Brussels sprouts are all from the mustard family. Eat only one from this family a day. Asparagus, onions and garlic are all from the lily family. Beets, spinach, and chard are from the goose-foot family. Carrots, parsley, and celery are from the parsley family. Lettuce and artichokes are from the composite family. Beans and peas are from the legume family. Tomatoes are from the potato family. For a more detailed explanation see the chapter "Rotating Your Foods" in this book. (Note: The lettuce talked about here is only the loose leaf varieties such as Green Wave, and Red Sails lettuce. Loose leaf lettuce varieties are the only ones that should be considered for eating. Iceberg lettuce is not good for you and should be avoided.)

Some organic vegetables cost close to normal vegetables, and some are three times as much. BUT, it is worth it. Canned and frozen organic vegetables are also available. Watch for sales.

Eat vegetables raw, juiced, or cooked as little as possible to retain most of their nutrients. (Remember when you steam vegetables, bring the water to a boil BEFORE adding the vegetables.) Some vegetables are good cold and seasoned. One of my favorites is cold, cooked, broccoli with salt and a squeeze of lemon juice. Try your own combinations.

Vegetable soups are very nutritious and provide a nice variation to the vegetable preparation. There are several good cook books available with suggestions for vegetable soups.

To get the most benefit from vegetables, juice them. Juicing is a convenient way to consume vegetables in their raw, uncooked form, which retains the maximum amount of vitamins. Plain carrot juice is great, but many exciting juice combinations are possible. Dr. Norman W. Walker's book "Fresh Vegetable and Fruit Juices" gives many recipes and hints on getting the most from your juiced vegetables. As in cooking or eating vegetables raw, the end product is only as good as the starting ingredients. Fresh organically grown vegetables are going to give you the best juice.

If you can have your own organic garden, do it. Even if you live in an apartment, growing container lettuce, tomatoes and other compact vegetables is very possible. Also, it helps cut food costs. (Gardening is also a great stress reducer too!)

In Summary:

1. Eat ORGANIC vegetables if at all possible. It makes a BIG difference.

2. Choose vegetables that are not genetically engineered. We really don't know how safe altered vegetables are.

3. Green-leafy and non-starchy vegetables can be eaten with everything.

4. Eat at least two servings of vegetables at each meal, at least four servings a day.

5. Rotate the vegetables by families.

6. Eat vegetables raw, juiced, as soups, lightly cooked, or as left-overs.

7. Juiced raw vegetables offer the maximum nutrition and energy.

8. Steam vegetables in a stainless steel sauce pan with a stainless steel steaming basket. Remember to bring the R-O water to a boil BEFORE you add the vegetables to lock in flavor and the most nutrients.

9. Grow your own vegetables to cut costs, increase supply, and control quality.

Fruits

Go Organic!!! There is a big difference between organic fruit and the non-organic fruit. First off, you don't have to scrape the wax off of the fruit. (See waxy tomato comments in the previous section.) Also, the boxes they are shipped in usually do not contain undesirable preservatives. Select fruit that is not genetically engineered. The flavor is again MUCH better. Organic fruits come fresh, in cans, in individual servings, and frozen. It may take some hunting, but they can be found. Again, like organic vegetables, organic fruit, especially fresh organic fruit, cannot be found all year round nor in all places.

Rotate the fruits according to families. Apples, pears, and quince are all from the apple family. Prunes, cherries, peaches, apricots, nectarines, and almonds are all from the plum family. Raspberries, blackberries, and strawberries are in the rose family. Blueberries and cranberries are from the blueberry family. Figs are in the mulberry family. Grapefruit, oranges, lemons, tangerines, tangelos, kumquats, and limes are in the citrus family. Persimmons, kiwi, pomegranates, and dates are all by themselves.

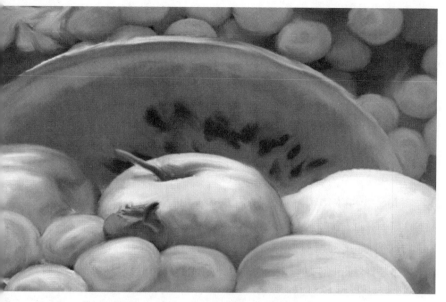

Fruits should be eaten alone as a snack and between meals. They digest better that way.

Fruits can be eaten raw, juiced, dried, cooked or in jams and jellies. Raw fruits are delicious. Organic assures no pesticides or wax coating on the fruit. If possible, grow your own fruit. Fruit juices are best served fresh and can be combined in many ways. "Fresh Vegetable and Fruit Juices" by Dr. Norman W. Walker suggests some fruit combinations. You can have fun creating your own, or copying combinations that you may have tried.

If you are eating dried fruit, make sure it does NOT contain any sodium sulfite or anything of a similar nature to preserve color or freshness, except lemon juice. Again, be careful that a good fruit is not ruined by the addition of undesirable chemicals. Purchasing quantities of organic fruit when it is least expensive and drying it is a good way to cut the cost of dried fruit and control the additives. Note: When eating a dried fruit, it is very easy to consume more than a normal serving. For example, a person may eat only eight fresh cherries at one sitting. However, they may eat a handful of dried cherries not realizing that the handful is the equivalent of 20 cherries.

Cooked fruits may be sweetened by adding apple juice if desired. If you purchase jams and jellies, make sure that they are all organic fruit with no added sugars.

In Summary:

1. Buy ORGANIC fruit if at all possible.

2. Select fruit that is not genetically engineered.

3. Rotate the fruits according to families.

4. Eat fruit alone as a snack.

5. Eat fruit raw, juiced, dried, cooked, or as jams and jellies.

6. Be sure that preservatives such as sodium sulfite are not added to enhance the color.

7. Dry your own fruit to save money and control additives.

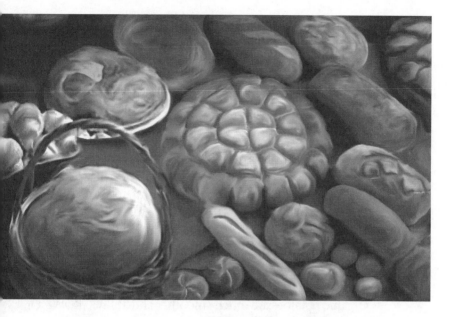

Starches

Combining foods to be digested quickly puts starchy foods in a separate category by themselves. Starchy foods should be eaten alone or with green leafy vegetables. (If you don't believe me, remember how full and miserable you felt during the holidays when you ate corn, bread stuffing, yams, potatoes, and pie all at the same time? Remember too, how long you felt stuffed?) I use my starch category foods as my breakfast and as snacks. (See chapter on "Food Combining" for more details.)

Some foods in this group include potatoes, yams, breads, grains, winter squash, cereal, rice, pasta, chestnuts, and peanuts.

Again, choose starches that are not genetically engineered. The grains seem to be one of the most heavily genetically engineered food types. Almost 50% of all corn, soy, and canola, grown in the United States and Canada are genetically engineered. So, choose ORGANIC. There is such a BIG difference. There is really no comparison. Organic starches are probably the easiest to find and available in the most variety of any of the organic foods. Again, dad really ate a lot more starches when they were organic than he would the non-organic kind. They even have SUPER organic French fries available!!

Organic potatoes are much smoother and THEY GROW! Or, haven't you noticed? Most bags of potatoes in the regular grocery stores now-a-days WILL NOT GROW if you plant them. They have been treated to kill them so they won't sprout in the refrigerator. ORGANIC potatoes WILL grow. Potatoes are in the nightshade family, as are tomatoes and eggplants. Try to avoid eating these three together.

Yams and sweet potatoes are from the morning glory family, while pumpkin, and other winter squash are from the gourd family.

Breads are a really big change as most people are used to eating wheat or whole wheat bread. Again, a good health food store will have breads made with alternative grains. Bread that is 100% rye is usually easily available. Some more alternative grains are millet, spelt (which contains gluten), quinoa, amaranth, rice, barley, and oats, just to mention a few. The flour from all of these grains is also available to do your own baking. Just become a good label reader. Some breads may have whole wheat in them, or honey or other things that you need to be careful with. Some breads are better toasted, and others are best with just butter.

There are many cereals available at most health food stores. If you are sensitive to honey, stay with the fruit juice-sweetened ones. When the label of a health food brand cereal says "oats, and apple juice", or "rice, and fruit juice", it really makes an impact when compared with other cereals that say "corn syrup, oats, sucrose, salt, and malt". One grain and fruit juice compared to one grain, three sugars and salt? The choice, to me, is simple. For dad, if he ate a regular store cereal, it would put him into bed for the rest of the day. If he ate a health food cereal, it would give him lots of energy.

Pastas are another category that is easy to replace with alternative grains. There are several brands of 100% rice spaghetti, lasagna, noodles, and macaroni, that when cooked correctly (boil hard for the entire cooking time) even fooled dad, a full-blooded-first-generation American ITALIAN. There is also great frozen pizza crust available.

Again, as with all other foods, rotate your grain/starchy foods preferably in a four day cycle. For example, one day have spelt, one day oats, one day potatoes, one day rice, one day barley, one day rye. If you do not have enough variety of grains in your diet for one week, or don't like some of the replacements, eat two grains a day. For example, I have millet and spelt on one day. Quinoa and potatoes on the next, etc.

In Summary:

1. Eat starches alone or with green leafy vegetables.

2. Buy ORGANIC if at all possible.

3. Buy grains, potatoes, and other starchy foods which are not genetically engineered.

4. Rotate the grains in a four day cycle.

5. Eat alone for breakfast or use as a snack.

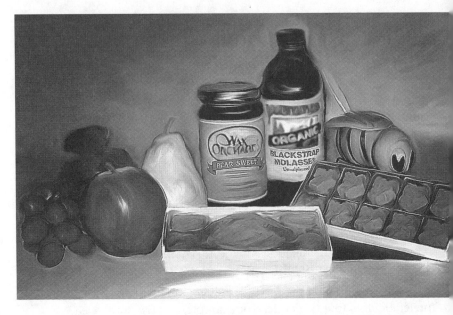

Sugars & Sweeteners

Sugars are the most quickly absorbed form of energy for the body. They can also be one of the trickiest too. If you are diabetic or know someone who is, you are probably aware of how fast blood-sugar levels can rise and fall. How many of us too, have grabbed a quick pick-me-up in the form of a candy bar, soda, or other sugar-loaded food. Sometimes it seems that we are a society that is run on sugar energy. While an occasional sugar pick-me-up may be all right, living on constant sugar energy is not good for your health.

As you start to eat better meats/proteins, fruits, vegetables, and grains, and use them and their energy as your main source of energy, you can eliminate almost all of the extra sugars in your diet and usually feel much better, be much healthier, and have better energy.

But for what little extra sugar you do consume, what kind of sugar you use makes a big difference.

All sugars are NOT created equal. All sugars contain 6 carbon atoms, 12 hydrogen atoms, and 6 oxygen atoms. But it makes a BIG difference what the bonds in the molecules are attached to, where they are attached, and how they are bent. From a chemist's point of view, a sugar is a molecule that is not flat or two-dimensional, but is three-dimensional. This bonding, bending, and arrangement of atoms and molecules gives us different types of sugars such as dextrose, fructose, glucose, lactose, maltose, and sucrose. Because of these different types of bonding, some sugars are rapidly burned, some burn less rapid and some sugars are completely ignored by the body. Therefore, a person may not be able to handle a sucrose as well as a fructose, or a lactose.

Dextrose is a very widely used sugar and is more commonly known as corn sugar. Corn sugar is most often listed on labels as "corn syrup." This sugar is not only used in foods such as bacon, breads, cereals, pastries, candy, catsup, cheese, chow mein, jellies, processed meats, peanut butter, and sherbet, to name a few, but is also in items such as sticking tape, aspirin, and plastic food wraps.

Fructose naturally occurs in fruit and honey. Fructose is absorbed more slowly than other sugars and has less of an effect on blood sugar levels than other sugars even though it can be twice as sweet as sucrose.

Glucose occurs naturally in blood, grapes, and corn sugar. Glucose is sweeter than sucrose and is used in sausage, hamburgers, and other prepared meats. It is used to treat diabetic comas and other nutritional conditions.

Lactose is milk sugar, present in the milk of mammals. It is interesting to note that cow milk reportedly contains about 4.3 percent lactose, while human milk contains about 6.7 percent.

Maltose is malt sugar, which comes from malt extract. Malt extract comes, most often, from barley. After preparation, the malt can be used as a nutrient or in cured meat and poultry.

Sucrose is cane sugar. It is probably one of the most widely used sugars today. In a country concerned about its weight, it is interesting to note that it has been reported, sucrose actually encourages fat production in the body.

So, if you are allowed sweeteners on your diet, which ones are the most healthy? Which ones do you use?

Refined white sugar, brown sugar, corn syrup, and commercially prepared fructose are definitely in the do NOT use category. These refined sugars have all of the vitamins and minerals refined out of them and have been classified by health enthusiasts as fast burning, empty caloried sugars that have been clinically linked to diabetes, obesity, cardiovascular disease, and are probably responsible for those unhealthy sugar highs.

Another sweetener NOT to use is aspartame. This sweetener has been controversial since its accidental discovery in 1965. When the discovering company asked for FDA approval in 1973, it took many years of extra research before finally being approved in 1981 over many serious objections by neurologists and others.

Aspartame is made up of aspartic acid and phenylalanine.

Aspartic acid itself has no known toxicity, but some reports claim that aspartic acid can convert into aspartate.

Aspartate is known to cause nerve cell damage especially in infants and children. It should also be avoided by others with neurological damage.

Phenylalanine in very high doses, it has been reported, may cause lower levels of serotonin and may lead to depression. Phenylalanine taken by people who have the genetic disorder phenylketonuria (PKU) may experience seizures and schizophrenia, and may be the source of some mental problems in children.

Other studies have shown that when aspartame is heated above 86° F (30° C) it breaks down into methanol and formaldehyde.

Methanol, which is known as wood alcohol, is extremely poisonous causing blindness and death even in small amounts.

Formaldehyde not only causes cancer, but is known to interfere with DNA replication and causes birth defects.

In 1984 the Arizona Department of Health Services became concerned at the high levels of methanol in aspartaine products in Arizona. The aspartaine breakdown temperature of 86 degrees F is easily exceeded during Arizona's 110 degree F summers. Temperatures are often over 150 degrees F in uncooled vehicles. However, the FDA decided that the levels found were "within tolerable levels" and "within standards."

But, other countries such as Mexico have placed warnings on products containing aspartame to notify the people of these possible dangers.

If aspartame is stored a long time or is heated, it breaks down into diketopiperazine (DKP). Once it is inside the body, DKP is reported to raise cholesterol, increase uterine polyps, and increase stomach cancer.

In addition to this, The National Cancer Institute has noticed a 67% increase in brain tumors between 1973 (first year aspartame wanted approval) and 1990 in people over 65. Brain tumors in all age groups are up by 10 %.

Seizures have been traced to aspartame by Massachusetts Institute of Technology. Airline pilots are not to use aspartame products before flights because of the seizure risk as reported in several Aviation trade magazines.

Even the American Diabetes Association (ADA) has noted that evidence links major problems in diabetic control to the use of aspartame. These problems range from "leading to clinical diabetes", and "poor diabetic control", to aggravating conditions such as retinopathy, cataracts, and neuropathy. In Mexico, a warning on the label of aspartame containing products states that the products are not to be used by a diabetic unless approved by a physician.

A 1994 report of the Department of Health and Human Services documents over 90 different symptoms and possible reactions to aspartame. These include headaches, seizures, depression, fatigue, weight gain, irritability, insomnia, memory loss, and joint pain.

Conditions that were triggered or got worse by using aspartame include brain tumors, multiple sclerosis, epilepsy, alzheimer's, Parkinson's disease, ADD (attention deficit disorder), chronic fatigue syndrome, fibromyalgia, and diabetes. There are claims of aspartame causing increased thirst and as a result you drink more aspartame products thus consuming more aspartame and creating a greater risk of problems. There are even some reports of deaths caused by aspartame.

In summary, the risks are too great to use any aspartame product even in small FDA approved amounts.

So, which sweeteners can you use?

Good sugars are ones which are natural, not refined, and therefore contains vitamins, minerals, and other nutrients essential for good health. These sugars are metabolized more slowly in the body giving the person a more even blood-sugar level. This is in addition to the natural vitamins and minerals a person needs.

The most common natural sugar is probably the fructose found in fruit.

Other naturally sweet foods are winter squashes, sweet potatoes, yams, and carrots. Remember the natural sweetness of carrot cake and cookies made with pureed squash?

In addition to these natural fruit and vegetable sugars, there are several other acceptable sugars.

Anasake is a Japanese drink made from rice. It is easily digested and the glucose and maltose in it burns slowly and evenly in the body.

Barley malt syrup is made from whole sprouted barley. It is about half as sweet as molasses. It is mainly maltose with some glucose and other simple sugars in it. It also contains B vitamins and protein.

Brown rice syrup is from brown rice and sprouted barley. This sugar is similar to barley malt syrup and contains maltose, glucose, some complex carbohydrates, minerals, and B vitamins.

Date sugar is made from dates. This sugar contains iron, potassium, other minerals and vitamins.

Dehydrated organic sugar cane juice differs from refined white sugar in the fact that it is dried and not refined. By drying, the minerals, vitamins and other nutrients remain with the sugar and are not stripped away by the refining process. This sugar is almost all in the form of sucrose. Be cautioned though, this kind of sugar needs to be organic. If not organic, the drying process concentrates the pesticides and herbicides used in the fields to grow the sugar cane. "Sucanat" is the usual short-hand name for this sugar.

Fruit juice concentrate is made by evaporating peach, pear, pineapple, grape or a combination of juices. This leaves mainly sucrose and some fructose as available sugars. This kind of sugar would have nutrients, minerals and vitamins similar to the fruits they were made from. Be aware though, that if you are allergic to some of the fruits, you may not be able to use this kind of sugar.

Granular Fruit Sweetener is composed of grape juice concentrate and rice syrup. It is a little less sweet than refined white sugar and contains slightly less than half of its sugar in the form of complex carbohydrates. This sugar is a good combination of fast and slow burning sugars. It also contains many vitamins and minerals.

Honey is a combination of glucose- and fructose- type sugars and contains some vitamins, minerals, enzymes, and pollen. It is sweeter than white refined sugar and is quickly absorbed into the blood stream. The best, most nutritious honey is honey that is processed with low heat and minimal filtration. Since honey is collected from flower nectar, there are many different kinds of honey. Be cautious if the honey is made from something you are allergic to. For example, if you are allergic to alfalfa, be cautious with alfalfa honey. Choose a honey from flowers you are not allergic to. *Note: Do not give honey to children under one year of age. It has been known to cause botulism in infants.

Maple syrup is mainly sucrose and is less sweet than refined white sugar. It is metabolized similarly to white sugar, but it has some calcium and iron in it. Buy only pure organic maple syrup. "Maple flavored" syrup contains corn syrup and may contain artificial coloring and flavoring. Non-organic syrups may contain formaldehyde or other chemical anti-foaming agents and mold inhibitors.

Molasses is the sweet syrup that is left when the sugar crystals are removed in the sugar refining process. Molasses is less sweet than white sugar, but contains calcium, iron, and B vitamins. Molasses needs to be organic and unsulfured. Non-organic molasses may contain pesticides and sulfured molasses may contain sulphur dioxide which is not only a problem for people with sulfur sensitivities, but is a toxic substance used to bleach vegetables and preserve fruits and grain and is known to destroy Vitamin A in preserved foods.

Sorghum syrup is made from sorghum, a cereal grain, similar to millet. This syrup is mainly sucrose and is a little less sweet than white sugar. It contains B vitamins and minerals.

Stevia is a sweetener that comes from the "yerba dulce" or "sweet leaf" plant native to Paraguay and Brazil. This sweetener can be hundreds of times sweeter than sugar. However, even though it tastes sweet, it is a sugar our bodies can't use, so it adds no calories and it does not affect blood sugar. Recently though, the FDA has questioned the safety of Stevia and has started to restrict it from the market.

In Summary:

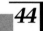

1. Eliminate all sugars that are refined.

2. Eliminate all corn sweeteners.

3. Eliminate all aspartame and other artificial sweetened foods and drinks.

4. Use only natural, unrefined and where possible, organic sugars.

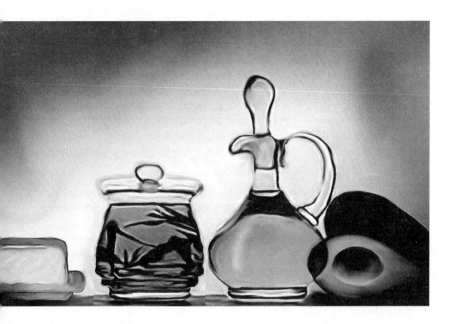

Fats
fats, oils, butter, avocados, and nuts

Fats are the most concentrated source of food energy. Fat molecules are larger than sugar molecules and typically burn slower than sugar.

In recent years, there has been a lot of concern about the amount of fat in American's diets, especially with the increasing overweight problems of all age groups. "No-fat" and "low-fat" have become popular not only in foods, but also in diet fads.

However, the body needs some fat to survive as there are some essential vitamins, like A, D, E, and K that dissolve only in fats. So, what are you to do?

When you change your eating habits and choose lean meat, chicken, fish, and start eating more vegetables and fruit, one's body tends to adjust to get more energy from the good sources of food. By switching to natural sugar products as outlined in the previous chapter, the body tends to adjust itself to tolerate the needed amount of fat.

It is interesting to note that many fat-free and low-fat foods, and diet drinks contain many fast burning sugars so when a person eats or drinks them, they can feel more energetic. (Remember how you have always heard that sugar will give you a quick pick-up?) But, if the body is burning the quick burning sugars, when does the body burn the larger fat molecules? It is ironic that these fat-free and low-fat products were probably being eaten in the first place to help the person loose fat, yet with so much sugar in them, the purpose is being defeated.

So, by eliminating all of the unhealthy sugars and other unhealthy foods in your diet and switching to healthy ones, quite often the desired weight loss occurs. You are able to eat the required amount of fats that your body needs.

I, myself, lost 15 pounds and have easily maintained my weight and energy for the last 15 years. Others that I know who wanted to lose more, have gradually taken off as much as 50 pounds in one year and have kept it off as long as they continued to eat healthier foods. They too felt a lot better and were more energetic, not only from weighing less, but from generally feeling healthier.

So, which fats? Again, there is a big difference between fat and oils not only in how they are processed, but in the kind of fat and oils that they are. First, pick a fat or oil that is liquid at room temperature. Oils on the whole are better for you than solid lard or margarine.

Next, choose a natural oil rather than a processed one. Naturally occurring oils have cis-controlling molecules on the same side of the molecule. Processed oils have trans-controlling molecules on opposite sides of the fat molecule. It is well known that trans-fatty acids and hydrogenated oils are dangerous and have been linked to high cholesterol, obesity and general poor health. One report even stated that the natural cis type fats and oils are half-used in the body on an average of only 18 days while trans type fats and oils take an average of 51 days for the body to half-use. So you want to be selective when you do use fats and oils.

Cold processed and expeller pressed are the best oils as processing can turn a good cis oil into a bad trans oil. Other good oil signal words are monosaturated, polysaturated, and low in saturated fat. Bad oil signal words are hydrogenated, partially hydrogenated, and saturated fat.

You also need to find a oil that you are not allergic to. Olive oil is probably the best naturally occurring oil to use. Canola oil is good only if it is organic. A lot of the non-organic canola oil today is made from genetically engineered seed and should be avoided.

Vegetable oils often have corn, soy, cotton seed, or peanut oil in them which can create major allergy problems for those sensitive to these ingredients. Cotton seed oil can cause severe allergy reactions. It is quite often genetically engineered.

For butter, use real organic butter. Organic butter assures no hormones or antibiotics have been given to the cows and therefore will not be present in the butter. Even with milk allergies, butter can sometimes be safely eaten because it comes from the cream part of the milk.

If you have to use a margarine, check carefully that it does not contain any oils that you are allergic to, or canola oil that maybe genetically engineered.

Avocados are also considered a fat food even though they are technically a fruit. An Avocado by itself for a snack gives me plenty of energy.

Most nuts and nut-butters are fat foods. Many times I will have a snack of a half of cup of cashew, almond, or other nut-butter. Great energy. (And no, I don't gain weight when I eat nuts this way. Another common dieting myth down the tubes.)

When planning your meals, fats and fat foods are best eaten with green leafy/non-starch vegetables, or by themselves.

Since we have been programmed to count things that we eat (calories, fat grams, etc.), if you feel the need to count something, count carbohydrate grams. Carbohydrates are monosaccharides and disaccharides or, in plain English, sugar and starch energy. If you are interested in losing weight, limit yourself to 100 grams of carbohydrates a day with most of the grams coming from complex carbohydrates such as vegetables and fruits, and very little from simple carbohydrates such as sugar, starches, and refined grains. To maintain weight, eat about 200 grams a day. For more information, there are several books and articles available on carbohydrates and addiction to carbohydrates.

In Summary:

1. Choose oils that are cold pressed, monosaturated, or unsaturated.

2. Do NOT use oils that are hydrogenated or partially hydrogenated.

3. Use fats such as butter, olive oil, avocados, and nuts for energy.

4. Eat fats alone or with green leafy/non-starch vegetables. (Butter on bread is okay though.)

5. If you have to count something, count grams of carbohydrates. (To lose weight, limit yourself to 100 grams a day).

6. Choose complex carbohydrates such as vegetables and fruits rather than simple ones such as sugar, starches, and refined grains.

7. Choose organic oils.

8. Do not use oil (especially canola oil) that may be genetically engineered.

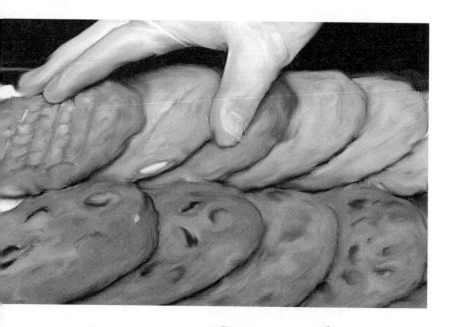

Snacks, Condiments, Herbs, and Spices

There are many snacks available if you get hungry during the day. First of all, try to eat something to fulfill the three meals a day eating routine as outlined in the sample menu at the end of this book. If you are still hungry, try some of the following. Just make sure that you eat them by themselves and just one serving.

- Fruit.

- Nut butters (peanut, almond, pecan, cashew, etc.)

- Any of the starch category items by themselves.

- Cookies (There are many wheat-free and fruit juice sweetened ones that are super.)

- Ice cream products made with rice. Many flavors are available in bars and quarts.

- Energy bars. Check carefully, but there are some really good ones that have only fruit juice as sweetener and are very delicious. Even stay away from those with several natural sugars.

- Applesauce.

- One cup of pudding. It's really good! (A commercial rice-based pudding even tastes just like lemon pudding and butterscotch pudding. They have done a really good job.)

There is a growing number of excellent condiments out there that are really good substitutes for things that we use every day. Catsup, mustard, mayonnaise, pickles, relish, olives, salad dressing, barbeque sauce, and salsa, just to mention a few, are available. Just make sure that you read the labels. Even jams and jellies are very well made. Again, choose organically grown products which are fruit-juiced sweetened and those with no sugars, no corn sweeteners, or artificial sweeteners in them.

For edible herbs and spices and food flavorings such as garlic, oregano, and pepper, again go to a health food store to purchase them. If organic are available, purchase those. Read labels carefully and select spices that are pure, natural, and have no added ingredients to preserve color or flavor (like they have in some cayenne pepper powders), or free-flowing agents. Some herbs you can grow on your window sill, or purchase fresh and then dry your own. Just make sure that the herbs are organic if purchased fresh.

Most pure organic herbs and spices can be used as seasonings as your diet restrictions allow and your body tolerates. You need to be aware though, that some herbs and spices may not be tolerated or may make you not feel as well. So use only the ones that work for your body.

Anciently people knew how herbs and spices added flavor to food. But before modern medicine, they used some herbs and spices as their only treatment for ailments. For medicinal use of herbs, contact a health care professional that is trained in herbs. Some herbs are very powerful medicine and should be treated as such.

One flavor enhancer that probably everyone needs to avoid in all forms though, is monosodium glutamate or MSG.

MSG is a compound that was isolated in 1908 from the Kombu (Laminaria Japonica) or sea tangle seaweed which was being used as a flavor enhancer in the Orient. It was embraced for use in the United States in 1948 by the major food companies. By 1968 serious questions to its affects were being raised.

Research has shown that MSG has a drug-like effect in that almost everyone will react to it at a high enough dose. Those who are sensitive to it will react to even trace amounts of MSG.

Reactions to MSG was once dubbed "Chinese Restaurant Syndrome." Research has shown that widespread use of MSG in food, (estimated 120 million pounds a year in the U.S. alone), may affect over 50 million people here in the United States. In almost all of the studies, a noticeable reaction occurred in over 1/3rd of the test subjects. Reported symptoms included migraine headaches, mild to severe depression, asthma, irritability, dizziness, diarrhea, chest pressure, heart arythmia, ADD, ADHD, PMS, prostrate trouble, rage, arthritis, rashes, slurred speech, nausea, and confusion, just to name a few.

Because MSG acts as a nerve toxin, researchers have started analyzing possible links between MSG and Alzheimer's, Parkinson's disease, ALS (Lou Gehrig's disease), and Huntington's disease. Also, because of possible links to neurological problems, victims of stroke, brain injury, and other neurological damage should avoid any and all use of MSG.

MSG can be listed on the label as "MSG", "natural flavoring", "hydrolyzed vegetable protein" (which contains up to 40% MSG), "spices", "natural seasonings", "autolyzed yeast", "yeast extract" (10-20% MSG), "flavoring", "sodium caseinate", "calcium caseinate" (approx. 12% MSG), or "Kombu" as seaweed or extract.

MSG can be found in products listed as "all natural" and even in organic products. It can be hidden in seasoning salts, flavor packets, broth (vegetable, chicken, or beef), bouillon, meat tenderizers, seasoning mixes, or flavor enhancers. Avoid premixed spices, garlic salt, and onion salt. Low-fat and fat-free items may contain flavor enhancing MSG as most of the item's original flavor was likely contained in the fat which has been removed. In fact, MSG can be found in almost all processed, canned, prepackaged foods as well as in fast food and restaurant foods. It is found even in health food and natural food markets. MSG is practically unavoidable. But, as a general rule of thumb, the more processed the food, the more likely it contains MSG.

In Summary:

1. Try to eat three meals a day before snacking.
2. If you have to have a snack, choose wisely.
3. Eat only one serving.
4. Use organically grown condiments.
5. Use condiments with no added sugars and that are only fruit juice sweetened.
6 Choose herbs and spices with care. You may react negatively to any herb or spice as well as any food item.
7. Use herbs and spices that are organic and have no preservatives or free flowing agents in them.
8. Avoid MSG (monosodium glutamate). It is found in more foods than just Chinese food. Remember MSG can be hidden as "Kombu", "flavor enhanced", "natural flavoring", "hydrolyzed vegetable protein", "natural seasonings", among other names. Also the more processed a food is, the more likely it contains MSG in some form.
9. For medicinal herbs, contact a professional trained in herbs.

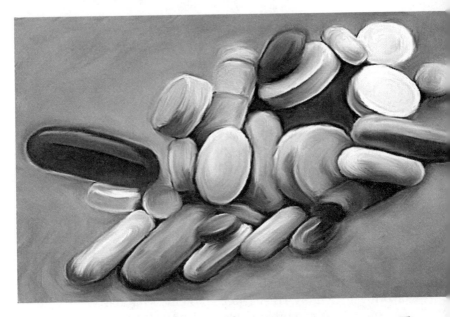

I am grouping these things together because they fit together.

Salt, Minerals & Vitamins

First off, still use salt. Salt is essential for the human body to live. There is salt in blood and tears, and the correct amount of salt is essential for the cells in the body. Salt also helps the body digest grains, fats, and oils. Salt is also essential for proper nerve and muscle function. Additional salt has even been suggested for those with Chronic Fatigue Syndrome to help relieve symptoms.

However, there is a very BIG difference in the

kind of salt used. Salt, as most people know it, is sodium chloride or NaCl. But to a chemist, salt can be one of dozens of compounds resulting from combining a mineral "acid" with a "base".

Table salt, which is found in most grocery stores, is highly refined. This refined salt is usually gathered by machines or drawn up in collection ponds by pumping water into a salt mine and then kiln drying the salty brine to eliminate the water. During the refining process, all of the trace elements that naturally occur in salt are removed which leaves the salt to government standards. When tested, this salt contains on the average 97.5% sodium and chloride. The other 2.5% is made up of additives such as a bleach to give the salt a fine, white look, stabilized iodine, and other additives to prevent the salt from absorbing water, which keeps it free flowing.

Many sea salts are taken from dry seabeds or sea water that has been sundried or processed. These salts have more of the natural occurring trace elements in them than refined table salt. However, analysis shows most sea salts contain on an average 98% sodium and chloride and only 2% of trace minerals as mineral salts. Again, the government standard limits the amount of naturally occurring elements in this sea salt. It usually ends up containing only 10 to 16 different trace elements.

The BEST salt to use is one that is collected from the sea, sun dried, and not up to government standards. This salt, on analysis, averages 84% sodium chloride and the other 16% anywhere from 36 to 84 trace minerals. Research has shown that the body needs most of these trace minerals to function. In fact, it has been proposed that the lack of some of these trace elements is having a major effect on Americans' health and supplementing them by taking mineral supplements is not the same as getting them naturally from salt.

Personally, I can really tell the difference in salt. Currently, I use a salt that contains 36 trace elements in it. I tried the other sea salts with only 10 trace elements in it and the energy and vitality was not there. In fact, now when I feel exhausted or run down, especially in southern Arizona's 100+ degree F summer heat, I will come in and take a sprinkle of salt on my hand and lick it. Within a minute or two, my energy is back.

A good salt crystal is cubic in form and about the width of the small wire loop on a regular paper clip. (About 3/16th of an inch- so you need to grind the salt before using it if it comes in "rock" form.) The best natural salt is gray in color, but still sparkles. Other salts that are not as good may look pink or other colors according to where the were mined. Pure white is the worst as this salt probably has been bleached and all of the trace minerals removed. The best salt will feel moist and will clump. This trait is an indication that the salt is probably sea salt recently sun-dried and has been stored properly. Yes, you will have to add a pinto bean to the salt shaker or tap the shaker to loosen the salt before using it, but that is a small price to pay for a good salt.

With the salt that I use that has 36 trace minerals in it, I don't seem to need any additional minerals except one, potassium, added to my diet. The salt seems to supply all of the ones that I need. So try the different salts and see if you can find one that supplies all of the trace minerals that you need. If you can't find one, then either let your body tell you which ones you need or consult a good health care professional who can balance extra minerals with those you are getting in your salt.

I can say the same about vitamins what I said about extra minerals. You should listen to your body and if you feel that you could use some vitamins, either try a few on your own, or consult a good health care professional that is knowledgeable with vitamins.

Note too, that all minerals and vitamins are not created equal. I had to search for years for a good potassium that my body liked. This potassium was compounded with three kinds of potassium where the other brands were only composed of one. It really made a difference. Again, listen to your body. If you need to take a supplement every day, do it. Sometimes it will only be once a week or twice a week. Let your body be your guide.

If you decide that you want to supplement your vitamin and mineral intake and want to try some on your own, stay with a good local health food store or market. The national chains tend to be watched by a person who is hired for the wage and is usually limited to general knowledge or the brands that the chain sells. A local or privately owned store will usually know their products better because giving the customer good advice will make or break their business. They will also have a larger variety of products to choose from than the chain store that must sell what the chain supplies or only the store brand.

In Summary:

1. Change your salt to one that is natural, sundried, contains many trace elements, and is from the ocean.

2. Avoid salt that is kiln dried, or bleached, or has most if not all of the trace elements removed.

3. Be aware that even sea salt can be kiln dried, bleached, or its trace elements removed.

4. The BEST salt is gray in color yet sparkles, is moist to the touch and clumps in the salt shaker. (Needs to be ground if it comes in rock form.)

5. Supplement minerals with the ones that your body tells you that you need after you have changed your salt.

6. Supplement vitamins with the ones that your body tells you that you need.

7. Purchase vitamins and minerals at locally owned health food stores rather than national chains.

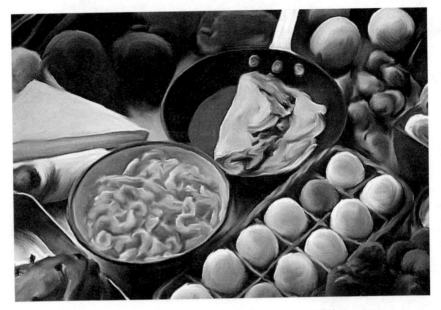

Food Combining

Food combining is a method of eating certain foods together and avoiding other combinations to improve digestion.

Research by physicians since the late 1800's has shown that the body has different times and conditions to thoroughly digest the food we eat.

The length of time to digest the food will be different for each individual, but averages for a normal healthy person have been determined. Proteins such as meat, poultry, cheese, and fish digest in 4 to 8 hours. Starches such as potatoes, bread, rice, and pasta take 3 to 4 hours. Fruits take 20-40 minutes. Vegetables take various times.

Proteins are mainly digested by the acids in the stomach. Starches start digesting in the saliva of the mouth. However, research has shown that when proteins reach the stomach, the enzymes from the saliva are neutralized. This results in the slowing of digestion of starches, thus taking them much longer to thoroughly digest. So, if a meal contains both starches and proteins, say meat and potatoes or bread, the digestion process slows way down and may take longer than the average eight hours.

Of course, the question is why should we care? The reason we should care is that slowing down or stopping the digestion of foods in the body has been shown to lead to many health problems. Food sensitivities, or allergies, arthritis, high cholesterol, heartburn, ulcers, constipation, sleep problems, stress, diabetes, and obesity are just some of the conditions that have reportedly improved when proper food combining has been followed. Proper digestion also allows the body to obtain the most nutrients and energy that it can from the foods we eat. So, it is very much to our advantage to properly combine our foods for maximum health.

When you are planning your menu, do the best you can to follow the proper food combining suggestions. If you find that you are still having some problems digesting your foods, you may want to add some digestive enzymes to your diet. These enzymes may be in tablet, capsule, or liquid form. Consult your doctor for some suggestions. If he or she does not have some to suggest, consult with a knowledgeable person at a health food store. Keep trying until you find the best combination that works for you.

There are several variations of food combining theory, but some divisions seem very standard. These divisions are summarized in the tables and charts that follow.

FRUITS-(acid, sub-acid, sweet, fat)

Acid and sub-acid fruits need to be eaten alone.

Sweet fruits may occasionally* be eaten with starches.

Avoid eating any fruit with proteins (except avocados).

Avoid eating any fruit with vegetables (except avocados).

*Occasionally means less than once a week. Preferably no more than twice a month.

PROTEINS-(complete, incomplete, fat)

Best eaten with non-starch vegetables.

May be occasionally eaten with starch vegetables.

Avoid eating with fruits (except avocados).

Avoid eating complete proteins with starches.

Incomplete proteins may be eaten with starches.

Fat proteins may be eaten with anything.

FATS-

Best with starch and non-starch vegetables.

May be eaten with anything.

VEGETABLES-(non-starch, starch, legumes)

Eat non-starch vegetables with proteins, fats, and starches.

Eat starchy vegetables with starches.

Starch vegetables may occasionally be eaten with proteins.

Eat legumes alone or with non-starch vegetables.

Avoid eating any vegetable with fruit (except avocados).

STARCHES-

Eat with non-starch vegetables or alone.

May eat with starch vegetables.

May eat with fats.

May occasionally eat with sweet fruit.

May occasionally eat with incomplete proteins.

Avoid eating with complete proteins.

Avoid eating with acid and sub-acid fruit.

Fruits

Eat alone	Okay with vegetables/proteins	Alone or Occasionally w/Starch
Acid	**Fat**	**Sweet**
Grapefruit	Avocado	Banana
Lemons		Dates
Limes		Figs
Nectarines		Grapes
Oranges		Raisins
Pineapples		
Tangerines		
Tomato		
Sub-Acid		
Apples		
Apricots		
Blackberries		
Cherries		
Currants		
Gooseberries		
Kiwi		
Mangoes		
Melons		
Papayas		
Pears		
Plums		
Raspberries		
Strawberries		

Proteins

Complete		Incomplete		Fat
Eat with non-starch vegetables/occasionally with starchy vegetables		*Eat with non-starch vegetables may eat with starchy vegetables*		*Eat with anything*
Beef		Dry Beans		Nuts
Cheese		Dry Peas		(except peanuts)
Eggs		Green Peas		Seeds
Fish (all)		Legumes		
Lamb		Lentils		
Milk		Peanuts		
Pork				
Poultry (all)		*Note:*		
Soy		*These incomplete*		
Yogurt		*proteins are also*		
		starchy vegetables.		

Fats

Best with vegetables
Eat with anything

Butter
Lard
Oil

63

Vegetables

Non-Starch	Starch
Eat with anything except fruit	*Eat with starches only occasionally with proteins*

Non-Starch	Starch
Artichokes (globe)	Corn
Asparagus	Green Peas
Beets	Jerusalem Artichokes
Beet Greens	Sweet Potatoes
Broccoli	Winter Squashes
Brussels Sprouts	Yams
Cabbage	
Carrots	
Cauliflower	**Legumes**
Celery	*Note: Legumes or pulses are*
Chard	*starchy vegetables and*
Cucumbers	*incomplete proteins.*
Eggplant	*Eat alone or with non-starch*
Endive	*vegetables.*
Escarole	
Garlic	Dry Beans (all)
Green Beans	Dry Peas (all)
Greens (all kinds)	Lentils
Herbs (all kinds)	Peanuts
Kohlrabi	
Leeks	
Lettuce (all kinds)	
Onions	
Parsnips	
Peppers	
Radishes	
Rutabaga	
Spinach	
Summer Squashes	

64

Starches

Eat with all vegetables & other starches or alone	Occasionally with sweet fruit
All Forms of Breads	**Sugars & Sweeteners**
cereals, flours, grains, & pastas:	
Amaranth	Barley malt
Barley	Honey
Buckwheat	Molasses
Kamut	Rice Malt
Millet	Stevia
Oats	Sugar
Quinoa	
Rice (all varieties)	
Rye	
Spelt	
Triticale	

In Summary:

1. Food combining allows for easiest digestion.

2. Good digestion allows maximum nutrition from the foods we eat.

3. Poor digestion has been linked to food allergies (sensitivities), arthritis, diabetes, heartburn, and obesity among other ailments.

4. If after properly combining your foods you still have problems with digestion, use some digestive enzymes.

5. Simplified Rule of Thumb for Food Combining:

    -Eat fruits alone

    -Eat proteins with non-starch vegetables

    -Eat starches with vegetables only

    -Sugars and sweeteners count as starches

    -Avoid eating starches with proteins

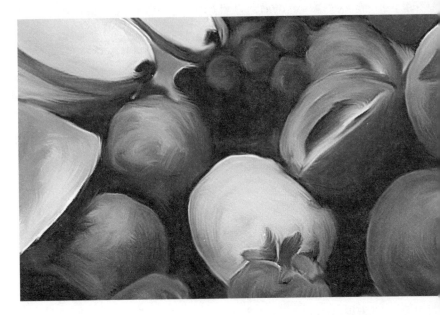

Rotating Your Foods

Ocne of the most useful techniques in living with food allergies is to rotate your foods.

Many doctors believe that some of the food sensitivities and allergies that are present today are as a result of improper digestion and eating the same foods everyday.

I know for myself, I cannot eat the same food more than once or twice in a twenty-four hour period. Yet, after three to four days, I can eat that food again with no problem.

So, to avoid a reaction by eating a food to often, you need to rotate them.

To rotate your food, you need to select your food from a different family each day for four days. After the fourth day, you can eat something from the same family again.

For example: For a protein, you would have a cattle family product on day 1, a poultry family product on day 2, a fish family product on day 3, and a legume product on day 4. Then after day 4, you would start the rotation over again. Cattle family product day 1, poultry day 2, fish day 3, and legumes on day 4, etc.

You would do the same for your vegetables, fruit, grains, oils, and sweeteners. (See creating your rotation diet in the section; "Making Your Menu.")

Some people can shorten their rotation times to only three days on some foods. Other foods you may have to have a 7day or longer period between eating them. Adjust your times according to how you feel. You know your body the best.

The amount of food you can eat will vary. Personally, I found that if I eat too much of one item either at one sitting or during the day, I will have to lengthen the time before I can eat it again. Sometimes just one more bite can be too much, so I have learned to save it for later, or toss it. So, be aware of the portion size you can eat.

Another thing you may have to watch for is eating two things from the same family at the same time. For example; Eggplant, tomatoes, and white potatoes are all from the potato family. I cannot eat tomatoes and potatoes at the same meal or during the same day. Eggplant with tomatoes doesn't work well either. So, be aware of too many items from the same family during one day.

In the Appendix, there is a list of plants and animals that are commonly eaten. Depending on what book, or if you are a biology major, the categories can be broken down into very small or very large categories. I have chosen to break down the categories into a level that I feel would be the most useful for an average person and most practical for this book. Note: some books put some items in different categories.

Use the food family list the Appendix with the charts in the chapter entitled "Making Your Menu" to complete your menu.

In Summary:

1. Eating the same food everyday is not good for your health especially if you have allergies.

2. Rotate your food on a four to seven day rotation period.

3. Choose foods from a different family each day of your rotation cycle.

4. Be careful of the portion size of your servings.

5. You may not be able to have two items from the same family on the same day.

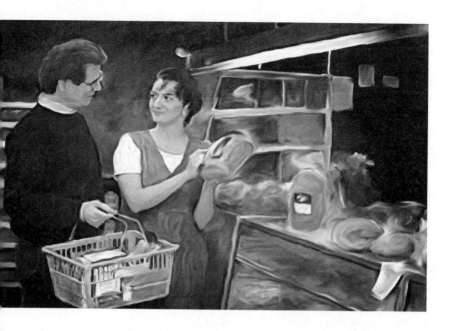

Where to Get All of This Stuff

Now that you have made the commitment to try this new and pure way of eating for at least one month, where do you purchase all of these things?

By now, you realize that the average chain food store that is across the nation or in a state will not be able to supply much, if anything at all, to eat or use in your new life style. I have found that some chain stores are starting to carry organic vegetables, fresh fish, and frozen organic vegetables, but you have to hunt for them. If you do find a store that carries organic foods, encourage these stores to continue to stock organic fresh and frozen vegetables by buying them, (they are often less expensive than speciality food stores), and commenting positively to the produce manager that you like to buy organic vegetables there. Stores will stock what consumers want and, most importantly, buy.

In my area and in a lot of cities, there are stores that are starting to cater to the person who wants to eat better. These stores usually have both organic and conventionally grown vegetables available since organic vegetables are not available at all times of the year. These stores probably will have a butcher-served meat counter and there are often notices that certify that the beef or chicken is hormone free. They will most likely have a fish counter. These stores will have a variety of canned goods and also a section with cereals, chips, natural soda, waters, and other safe foods and products. There are also many types of frozen foods that are available that would fit into a healthy diet.

If a local health food store does not have some of the items, ask if they can start carrying them or if they can special order items. Many stores will accommodate their customers and look on it as good business. The stores will carry what the customers want and buy. Just remember, they must sell their stock to keep in business so work with them.

The main thing to remember in any store is to read the labels and shop carefully. As has been mentioned before, the price will be the same to a lot higher at a health food store than at the regular store. You have to make the commitment to choose to buy better food and then follow through. Many of these stores do have sales and specials, and just like a good shopper in any store, watch and use the sales. Some stores will special order or give case discounts. Check prices at several stores. We get our toothpaste at one store (and that is all that we get there) because it is two to three dollars cheaper there than anywhere else. It can be done. When you get to feeling better, it will make every penny well worth it. (Not to mention the fewer doctor visits.)

For snacks and other baked goods, there are more and more allergy-free cook books available which have tested wheat-free, dairy-free, and other allergy-free baked goods. Sometimes good recipes are hard to find, but there are some good ones out there. Exchange recipes with friends.

Check some allergy-related web-sites for recipes and other allergy information on products. Many allergy-free products and/or healthy foods are available through the internet. Some bakeries will ship case lots to your house for a nominal shipping fee. Use caution in whom you deal with like you do for any other product or service bought over the internet.

If you have garden facilities available, grow as many things as you can. Not only can you control the fertilizer and pest control, but many times, you can stretch the growing season and pick fresh vegetables when they are not available in the stores or, if they are available, they are outrageously priced. (One year, I was producing tomatoes in January, by using frost protection cloth when organic tomatoes were selling for $5.99 a pound in the store. I really got paid back for my gardening effort then!!) A small two foot wide garden strip across the back does not take up much yard space and can yield a multitude of vegetables. Plant vegetables instead of flowers if space is at a premium.

Instead of planting ornamental trees, plant fruit trees. If the neighborhood has a code, plant the fruit trees in the back yard. It will take a couple of years to start getting a crop, but it will be worth it.

Choose trees that will grow in your climate. Even in the HOT Arizona heat, I personally have eight grapefruit, one orange, one tangerine, three varieties of pear, one peach, one persimmon, one pomegranate, and one pecan tree. I also have two grape vines and a 100 square foot organic vegetable garden. All are in a functional, well landscaped one-fifth of an acre. It creates not only a micro-climate of cool during the hot summer, but produces plenty for the family and enough to share. It can be done.

Container gardening can be productive and is great for patios or apartments. It may not yield all of the vegetables needed, but it can make a welcome addition to purchased vegetables.

Farmer's markets can be a good source of vegetables. However, many questions need to be asked like whether or not they use pesticides or chemical fertilizers. Some farmer's market produce is fresher than the stores, but may still contain many pesticides or chemical fertilizers.

Some organic farmers have started organic co-ops where a monthly or yearly fee is collected and then the farmer delivers a weekly selection of vegetables to those who are part of the co-op. Some co-ops are so popular that there are waiting lists to join.

There are more and more options to getting good and wholesome food whether you are in the heart of the city or in the country.

In Summary:

1. Change shopping habits to a store that sells organic products, foods, and health and beauty aids.
2. If the store does not have an item, ask if it can be special ordered or stocked in the future.
3. Make your own snacks.
4. Share recipes that you have found or developed.
5. Check the internet for sources for products and information.
6. Grow as many of your own fruits and vegetables as you can.
7. Use container gardening if space is small or temporary like in an apartment.
8. Shop farmer's markets. Be sure to ask questions as all produce may not be organic.
9. Join an organic produce co-op.

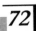

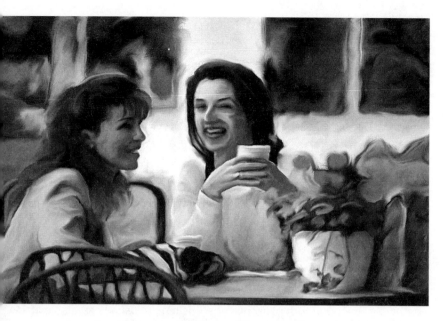

Lunches for Work *and What Do You Do At Social Occasions?*

For work and other times when you have to eat out, this new life style presents a challenge, but it is not insurmountable.

As you will see when you get to the sample menu, the meal the night before provides the left-overs for another day's lunch if you cook extra and plan ahead. Left-overs do not sound very appetizing, but they can be fixed to be very tasty. Some leftovers can be frozen and then thawed and warmed when needed, (but not by a microwave-oven.) Also, you don't necessarily have to go to the rabbit food look either in your lunches. A nice meat and vegetable combination is very easy to achieve and can be made to taste very good. (Yes, I have done sack lunches and dinners for many years. It can be done.) I have found that most people, when they question me about my "not eating something", or comment on my "interesting lunch," are very understanding when I tell them that I have food allergies.

In social situations, since eating is the national pastime for social events, try to choose the least offensive food when you are out eating.

Fresh seafood, plain beef, or chicken are usually available at most restaurants. More and more eating establishments are offering a larger variety of fruits and vegetables, either raw, in salads, or cooked. Salad bars are still great for fruit and salad fixings. A good server also has no problem with inquiries about possible allergic substances in the foods. They can even leave off added seasonings if MSG or other chemicals in the seasonings may be a problem. Just remember to tip them and/or the chef a little extra for their extra work.

For family and friend gatherings and other private, small social events, arrange with the hostess ahead of time for your needs when appropriate. Inquire in a tactful way about the menu and how things are cooked. Volunteer to bring some food to the gathering and then make sure you (as well as others) can eat and enjoy it. Don't expect the hostess to change the entire menu just for your needs. Eat a snack before you attend so you will not get too hungry, if needed.

For larger informal socials such as a church barbeque, bring a small lunch bag with your own barbeque items to eat with the other members of the group if you can. Some people may inquire, but most do not even notice when done quietly.

For situations such as an open house, eat before you go and enjoy visiting. With a plain glass of water in your hand and a lot of good socializing, most will never notice that you did not try the refreshments. Prepare an appropriate answer or other non-offensive statement in case you are questioned about trying the refreshments. Be as pleasant and truthful as you can, depending on the group.

If you are single, choose activities where you can bring your own food such as cookouts, hikes, and picnics as much as you can. Inform your date in a nice way about your needs. A good person to continue dating will be flexible and will be willing to meet your needs when they are presented in a nice way.

Remember, the less you make an issue out of what you need to eat, the less annoying it is to others and the more fun you will have. This is one case where the squeaky wheel sometimes does not get greased, but only left out.

In Summary:

1. Cook extra when you plan your night meal and use the left-overs for future meals and/or lunches.

2. For social situations, choose the best food you can, and enjoy yourself.

3. Inquire in a courteous way what the ingredients are or if a seasoning can be left off when ordering at a restaurant. Tip a correct amount.

4. Work with the hostess in small family and friend gatherings to meet your needs. Volunteer to bring something that you (and others) can eat.

5. For large, informal gatherings, quietly bring your own food that is similar to what is being served when you can. Eat before you go, if needed, then socialize and have fun.

6. Socialize while carrying a glass of water. Most will never notice you didn't try the refreshments.

7. If single, inform your date in a nice way about your needs. Choose "bring your own food" activities.

8. Don't make a big deal out of what you can and cannot eat. Be as pleasant as you can, eat what you can, and have fun!

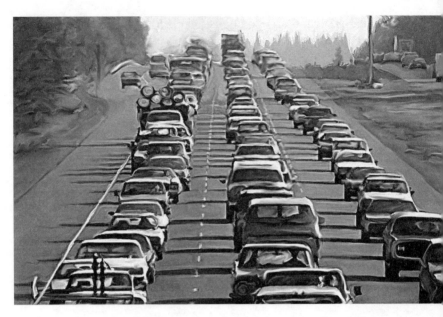

Other Potential Allergens in the Environment

There are other sources of allergens besides those in the foods you eat. Since many people have allergies to food have allergies to pollen, mold, and chemicals, it is to your advantage to be aware of other allergens you may come in contact with.

Soaps - For bath and hand. Soap daily touches the largest organ in our body, the skin. Many things are absorbed into the skin and physicians constantly use this fact in medical treatments using patches. Therefore, a good pure soap is important as a soap with added chemicals and dyes might allow unwanted chemicals to be absorbed into the skin. A plain castile soap is probably the mildest and gentlest soap that you can buy. It is available in a liquid or bar form. Castile soap is available plain, or with added ingredients such as lavender, oatmeal, vanilla or other scents in most health food stores and by special order in some major chain store pharmacies.

Soaps can be made with olive, coconut, or other oils. Try several and find the one that you like the best. Start with a plain unscented one, and then, when you have found a nice one, try adding the different scents. (Of course you could make your own. There are many books on making your own soap.) Most soaps available in the regular grocery stores still have many colorings, perfumes, fragrances, and dyes in them even though the industry has caught on to the natural movement and loves to plaster their products with the word "Natural" when they contain other ingredients that I would question as being natural!

Health and Beauty Aids - The very same things can be said about hair sprays, hand lotions, deodorants, tooth paste, shampoos, and other toiletries as has been said about soaps. There are many brands available that are more mild and pure than most brands that can be purchased in the regular stores. There are many deodorants that do a good job but without aluminum in any form. (There's that alzheimer's aluminum again.) There are also several brands of toothpaste that are great and have no extra sugars or bleaches in them. Hand lotion needs to be tried and carefully selected as even health food store brands can still create a rash or have other undesirable side effects. Most stores will have a tester bottle so you can try a product before you buy it. Remember too, that just because it is in a health food store doesn't mean that it is automatically safe for you as an individual. Try each product and find out which are best for you.

Aromatherapy - Be careful about the growing interest in aromatherapy. It has its place. But just like herbs, it should be under a person who is trained in the practice. This is especially true if you have asthma or other known allergies.

Scents, Perfumes, and Fragrances - In the selection of scents, perfumes, fragrances, and for men, after-shave and cologne, and the growing popularity of potpourri, be careful. Many people who are sensitive to food and other allergies can be allergic to scented items, even if they are all natural. If you are not sensitive to scented items, many commercial products contain chemical replicas of the natural world. There is a difference. Use natural and naturally occurring fragrances if anything at all. There are several books available on how to make and scent your own toiletries and potpourri with the fragrances that you like, and most importantly, toiletries and potpourri in which you can control all of the ingredients.

Clothes Detergents - Detergents and clothes dryer sheets for your laundry add chemicals to your clothes that can affect both your nose and your skin. Even the "Dye free, perfume free, dermatological tested" items that you can buy in the store may NOT be safe. (I know from sad experience.) There are many alternatives and the health store is only one place to try. Be cautious though. Health store detergents are not always safe for everyone. Try several and decide which is best for you.

Household Cleaning Products - Cleaning products for the dishes and home are another big area of toxicity and allergy irritation. Try several dish detergents and find the one that you like best. Hard water crust and soap scum in the bathroom and kitchen is no match for a half of a fresh lemon or grapefruit. It takes a little more elbow grease, but it is a lot safer. There are additional all-purpose cleaners available that are better and safer than those in regular stores. But again, all of these products are not safe just because you got them from the health food store.

Household Pests - Many natural alternatives are available for ants and other pests. Even if a product says that it is safe to use in eating areas and near food, doesn't mean that it really is. Many times I have noted the odor in "odorless" ant and roach baits. If you really think about it, they have to have some odor to attract the pest they are trying to get. I have been inside many houses where the people have put pesticide down and they claim that it is "odorless" or "It's gone now" and I can still smell it even months later. During June 2000, the EPA released a report on chlorprifos, a class of chemicals commonly known as Dursban. This report bans the use of chlorprifos in insecticides because of too high of risk of damage to the human brain and nervous system, especially in young children. Chlorprifos were originally developed as a deadly nerve gas by the Nazis during WWll and causes headaches, nausea, dizziness, seizures, and death. What is alarming is that chlorprifos have been widely used for the last 30 years as it is the most popular insecticide in use, replacing DDT. It has been estimated that it is being used in over 20 million homes and schools each year. For alternatives there are books available with suggestions to combat ants and other pests with natural items. One such ant remedy is to put cayenne pepper down where they are entering. One solution to ants getting into pet food on the floor is to float the pet food dish in a bowl of water (one dish inside another so they do not touch) since the ants will not swim across the water.

Garden Pests - Most garden pesticides contain chlorprifos which, as mention above, is too risky to continue using. Instead, pest control in the garden can be achieved with companion planting to ward off insects. (Yes, books are available on this subject too.) There are other tricks that can be used to get rid of insects. Yellow plastic plates smeared with petroleum jelly and hung in the garden does wonders for getting rid of pesky white flies. By using no pesticides, I often see birds wandering through the garden pecking the bugs off of the plants. The quality and quantity of food? Great! No problem with either quality or quantity. I have often picked a head of loose-leaf red lettuce that was 14 inches in diameter and 12 inches high and tender as you would ever want it. One beet was 15 inches in diameter and eight inches long. I consistently win State Fair awards on 19 out of 20 entries including Best of Class awards for my vegetables from my organically grown garden. This even in the next to impossible growing conditions of Phoenix, Arizona. It CAN be done!!

Car Products (Gasoline, anti-freeze, oils and other fluids)-If you live where there is a choice of gasoline with additives, try to use one that has alcohol- or ethanol- rather than M.T.B.E. (methyl-tertiary-butyl-ether) based smog control. Where I live, there is treated gasoline during the whole year to help control air pollution. The ethanol-based is a lot better for allergies and there is no appreciable wear and tear on the car engine. I've only had three tune-ups in 167,000 miles in my 1990 car and it runs fine with lots of power using the alcohol-based gas. Ethanol-based gas is also 5-10 cents cheaper per gallon here than M.T.B.E. gasoline. Also, I used to get really sick and would be really crabby and short tempered just after filling up with the M.T.B.E. gasoline. When I would come home and park in the garage, I could hardly breathe because of the exhaust and would end up with a headache. With the ethanol-based gas, I no longer get sick or crabby after filling up, and the garage gives me no more trouble after returning home. It really made a difference to me.

It is interesting to note that road rage goes up in the summer here when only M.T.B.E. is available and slows down in the winter when ethanol is also available. And didn't road rage increase about the time M.T.B.E. started to be added to the gas about 1991? And now that the truth has come out that warnings about M.T.B.E. were ignored and the effects of M.T.B.E. were not researched long enough, it really makes one wonder. It will be interesting in the next few years when more of the truth and hopefully more research will come out about M.T.B.E. Meanwhile, I know you can't control everyone else, but it does help to use ethanol-based gasoline when it is available.

Other car care products such as antifreeze are now being made more environmentally (and animal) friendly. Buy the products that are the best for the car and yet pay a good amount of attention to keeping the environment clean. By asking for more earth-friendly products, eventually the companies will listen. Even oil is easier to recycle today than it was years ago.

Indoor Air Pollution - This is a newly recognized source of environmental toxins which, now that people know what to look for, is more of a problem than once believed. Indoor air pollution can be caused by new carpets, the glue used in producing those new carpets, or the glue used in putting those new carpet down, formaldehyde in wallboards, out-gassing of paint, plastics, and furniture finishes, and other substances such as printer inks and copier toners. Other people in the same room may have smoked outside but the odor is still clinging to their clothes, or they may have perfume or after-shave on. Even the soap they use in their laundry can be annoying if it is something that you may be sensitive to. Some solutions are to have a good portable air purifier running near your work space, or asking building maintenance to circulate more fresh air. You could even tactfully ask co-workers if they would be willing to change a fragrance. For actual building problems, sealers have been created for carpets, walls, and floors that help create an environment that is acceptable. Even making a career change is something to consider if the change would solve the workplace problem. (And yes, I have been there and done that.) These are real world solutions to real world problems because sometimes a big change needs to be made and that is the only way to do it. It really helps to know too, that yes, this solution has been tried and a good life can and does go on after a major change. I personally changed careers three times. First, from a chemistry major (way too many chemicals there!!) Then, to teaching math at the junior college level (VERY contaminated building-even the Environmental Protection Agency inspected it, when seven out of nine of us instructors got very sick.) Then, to designing educational software and materials in a home office in order to control the indoor pollution as much as I needed to control it. It can be done!!

In Summary:

1. Change all health and beauty products to ones that are more pure and unscented, if necessary.

2. Change all cleaning supplies and laundry soaps to more pure ones.

3. Be a label reader. All that is marked "Natural" or "Herbal" or "Dermatological tested" is not automatically safe to use.

4. Beware and be aware of fragrances and scents in toiletries, home products, and as therapy.

5. Use natural means of pest control both in the garden and in the home.

6. Use ethanol-based gasoline and other car products that are more environmentally friendly.

7. Just because a product is sold in the health food store or is advertised as "Safe" it is not always safe enough. Try several.

8. Explore options if environment at work is causing allergy problems. Consider a career change if needed.

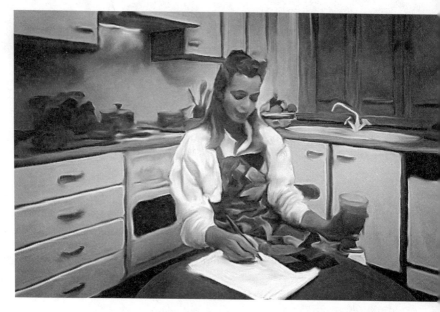

I've Decided to Change

Now, how do I do it?

Right now you may be feeling a bit overwhelmed with all of the differences in eating habits that have been presented in this book. It is rather a shock too, if you have been told that you MUST change your eating habits. It is a life-time of patterns that are hard to change. (Dad used to grumble at the table when Mom and I fed him good food. But, he soon enjoyed eating more and was much more healthy and quit grumbling.)

At first this new life style may seem too restrictive, but as you go along and make the changes, with the better energy that you feel, you may wonder why you didn't do this before. After changing my life style over 15 years ago, I don't really feel restricted or left out or denied any foods that I like. Most people look at what I bring for lunch and comment on how good it looks and some even look forward to finding out what I will be bringing for that day. Others comment on how they wish that they had the discipline to eat healthy the way that I do. As time has gone on, there have been good and acceptable substitutes for most of the foods I used to eat. It may take a while to fully implement the changes and feel good about them, but it is worth it!

If a doctor has recommended that you change your eating habits and has given you a list of foods and items to eat and those to avoid, use the list you have been given in the frame work of this book to plan and prepare your meals.

If you have not seen a doctor about changing your diet, it is wise to check with your physician before starting any dietary change. Please do so!

If you have checked with your physician and you have been okayed for a diet change, but was given no specific list to follow or very few items to avoid, you may want to consult one of several reputable food guides available in books to form your list of what to eat.

A couple of the best and most highly recommended books to read are "Eat Right 4 Your Type" and "Live Right 4 Your Type", by Dr. Peter J. D'Adamo with Catherine Whitney. The food suggestions given in these books are based on scientific evidence and have many years of proven success behind them. Their observations are based on blood type-A, B, AB, or O, which is fairly easy information for everyone to obtain. Many doctors, as well as many others in the health field, highly recommend these food guidelines to their patients.

Remember though, each person's body is slightly different. So even with a list from your doctor or a reputable book, you still need to listen to your body and if you have a problem with a certain food, don't eat it. And since our bodies change over time, your list may change from the list you start out with.

Another way to determine what you are allergic to, so you can form or check your list, is to muscle test each item before you eat it. Muscle testing or Kinesiology is an alternative-health type of technique that uses your body's own electrical and nervous system. The theory is that if an item that you are allergic to is brought into your body's electrical field or aura, it will disrupt the field.

Following are three ways to test. All you need is another person's help. Before you begin, you'll need to remove any quartz movement watches from yourself and your testing partner, as their frequency of vibration will interfere with the test. Also avoid testing near other items that are giving off energy such as cell phones, computers, T.V.s, radios, and microwave ovens that are in use.

The first way to test is to stand or sit with your right arm straight out from the side of your body at shoulder height. Have your testing partner push at your wrist and try with gentle pressure to push your arm down. Keep your arm straight. You should be able to resist the pressure. Then pick up or touch the item being tested, with your left hand. Your testing partner again tries to push your arm down using the same amount of pressure. Try to resist with the same amount of pressure. If your arm goes down, you are most likely allergic to that item. If your arm does not, it is most likely okay.

Although this technique has been used for decades, it may be new to you. Practice a few times with items you know you are not allergic to, and then with some you know you are allergic to.

The second way to test is identical to the first except that the right elbow is bent so the right hand is in front of the right shoulder, again shoulder high. The testing partner should try and push at the bent elbow. This method is good for those that may be in a more delicate condition such as an elderly person.

The third way to test is using the allergy acupressure points on the thumb and middle finger of the left hand. To test this way, touch your tips of the thumb and middle finger together. (You may stand, sit, or lay down.) Have your testing partner try and pull them gently apart while you gently resist. You should be able to resist. Then, you pick up or touch the item being tested. Have your testing partner try with the same amount of effort to pull your thumb and finger apart while you resist with the same amount of effort as before. If you can resist and keep your finger tips together, that item is probably okay. If not, you are probably allergic to it.

This third method is the best for the elderly or if you are discreetly testing something in a store.

Personally, I have been muscle testing for over 15 years. I first went to my doctor for a list from an allergy test. I was also taught how to muscle test. Then if there was a new item, like a cookie, with only one questionable ingredient in it, I will discreetly muscle test it before I buy it. I will also test old items that I may have eaten but did not feel too good after eating it. I have found out that for me, muscle testing is accurate about 95% of the time.

Muscle testing is a skill that needs to be developed. Some people can pick it up and do it fairly easily. Others may have a harder time doing it. If you feel uncomfortable with it, don't use it.

Once you have obtained your food list, either from your doctor, a reputable health book, or by muscle testing, proceed with the rest of this chapter and book.

Now, how to really do it! There are two ways that a dietary change can be accomplished.

One is basically cold turkey, when you clean out all of your old stuff and put the leftovers in the trash or give them to a friend or relative who doesn't mind opened boxes of cereal, partial bottles of shampoo or other items. This way can be a dramatic change and expensive. But the results are faster, and it is easier to start feeling good quicker and gives this new way of eating an honest test. In fact, most who make this change, do it this way and within a month they feel great. It really is the best way to make these changes. So, really try to do it cold turkey.

The second way is to phase it in. To phase in this new style of eating, finish up what you have in the bottles and refrigerator and as things run out, replace them with more healthy alternatives. Buy meat and vegetables instead of a frozen dinner. Buy at least organic tomatoes and fruit without the wax coatings so prominent in the stores. If you can't or don't want to make the change overnight, then go at it step by step, applying the following steps as soon as you can.

Steps for Change:

Step 1: Eliminate all products with added sugars, colors, flavorings or preservatives. Read the labels carefully.

Step 2: Eliminate the "Sinister Seven" of wheat, corn, sugar, milk, soy, chocolate, and yeast in all forms.

Step 3: Eliminate any other items that you seem to get a reaction from, or that you have been told that you are allergic to.

Step 4: Rearrange your eating habits to three meals a day with snacks in-between. Properly combine and rotate your foods eating only meat/protein and vegetables at lunch and dinner, leaving starches and fruits for breakfast and snacks.

Step 5: Change the way you cook. No microwaves ovens. Steam your vegetables. Use stainless steel, glass, or enamel cooking and baking utensils.

Step 6: Change to reverse-osmosis prepared water for all your added liquids. Eliminate all soda pop, especially ones containing aspartame. Eliminate all drinks that contain caffeine.

Step 7: Start buying organic every time you can find it.

Although this method is usually easier on the family and budget, by changing your eating habits this way, you might not feel as good as fast, as the last thing you change may be the item that is bothering you the most. By changing this way, it may take you as much as 3-4 months to feel better. However, do what is best for you. Just determine your plan of attack and follow through.

For some of you, it may mean learning to cook, ie. using some means of food preparation other than a microwave oven. But, go ahead and buy some cookware and a steamer basket and learn to cook.

Also, choose the best way that you like to keep record of your changes and plan your menus. If you like to plan detailed menus, do it. If you like to keep a food diary, do it. If you like to just have a beef, chicken, the fish pattern, then do it. Experiment until you find the way that you like to make the changes, plan your menus and then follow through. Change methods when you feel like it.

Following this section will be several different ideas for menu planning and record keeping. Since everyone is different, choose the one(s) that you like the best, or combine them, create your own. Do it the way that is best for YOU! (I currently use a combination of methods and keep changing it to fit my needs and wants.)

If you only feel a little better, keep at it and don't get discouraged. Some of these changes and getting to feeling better may only take a day or two when an offending food is eliminated, especially when done cold turkey. Other changes may take a few weeks or months to notice. And, don't worry about slip-ups. Do the best you can and enjoy the benefits of it. It becomes VERY easy to stay with your new good eating habits when after you have been eating healthy you decide to splurge and get an immediate headache or other annoying reaction to what you ate. Or, after a month or two of eating healthy, you realize that you don't feel as terrible as you used to.

Changing a lifestyle (and lifetime) of eating habits is a big change and will not happen overnight. Keep it up even if it does take years to change! You will reap great rewards. Our family did!

In Summary:

1. It is normal to feel overwhelmed. Changing a lifetime of eating habits takes time and commitment. But, you can do it!

2. Check with your doctor to make sure a dietary change is advisable.

3. Get your list of foods to eat and to avoid, either from your doctor (preferred), a good health book, or by muscle testing each item.

4. Decide to change by cold turkey or by using the given steps and phase the change in.

5. Record how you feel in the following Chart of Progress.

6. Make your menus using the guidelines in the following chapter.

7. Then DO IT, and enjoy eating again!

Chart of Progress

Record all of the data at the beginning of the week. Use a scale from one to ten, with ten being the best. (Make copies of the chart before using.)

	Week __	Week __	Week __	Week __
Energy				
Aches / Pains				
Headaches				
Itchy skin/rash				
Sleep habits				
Weight				
Cravings				
Sniffles				
Stomach Problems				

Note: Sometimes when you have changed your eating habits and then go back to your old eating habits, you notice a larger difference than when you just compare from week to week. This may be because from week to week, the change is slight and not too noticeable. But when you stop and go back to the old habits, the difference is immediate. For example, dad would seem to be just a little better, but when we would let him cheat and go back to his poor food habits, it would really make a noticeable difference in his health almost immediately.

89

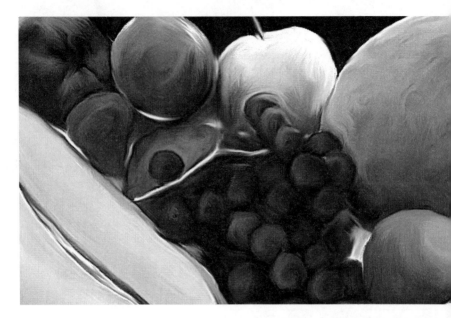

Making your Menu

Now: •You have decided to change. • You have your list of foods to eat and foods to avoid. • You have learned how to select your foods from the store. • You have learned how to cook your foods properly. • You have learned how to properly combine your foods. • You have learned how to properly rotate your foods.

Let's make your menu and do it!

Step 1: Look at the "Suggest List" section to refine your list of foods.

Step 2: Use the charts in the "My Rotation Diet" section to plan the rotation of your foods.

Step 3: Use the charts in the "Weekly Menu" chart section to plan your weekly menu.

Step 4: Happy Eating!

Note: For those of you who would rather use a "Check-Off Chart "or a "Written Menu" instead of a grid-type chart, use those sections instead.

Suggested List

The "Suggested List" is a list of grains, meats, proteins, vegetables, fruits, sweeteners, drinks, snacks, and other foods that are suggestions to answer the questions of "What Do I Eat?" Most of us may have gotten into a rut by cooking and eating the same vegetables, meats, or grains all of our lives. To all of a sudden have to eat a different grain each day for four days is a challenge when we may be familiar with only two or three grains. So, the "Suggested List" is exactly what its title says, a list of grains, meats, fruits, and vegetables, and other food items that you may or may not be familiar with.

Directions:

Step 1: Locate the pages which are titled "Suggested List, "Suggested List Example", and "Suggested List" which is blank.

Step 2: Photocopy the pages which are titled "Suggested List", and "Suggested List" which is blank as needed.

Step 3: Look over the "Suggested List". You can either:

Choice A: Follow the directions at the top right hand corner of the page by circling the items you tried and seem to have no reaction to, cross off the list the items you tried and cannot use or know you are allergic to, put a "S" by the items that you have had a small reaction to and still want to eat, and put a "?" by

Date _____/_____/_____

Grains	Meat/Protein	Meat/Protein	Vegetable	Vegetable

0-Circle the items you tried and seem to have no reaction to
X-Cross off the list items you have tried and can not use
S-The items that you had a small reaction to, but okay
?-The items that you are not sure of.

Fruit	Sweetener	Drinks	Snacks	Other

Date _____/_____/_____

Grains	Meat/Protein	Meat/Protein	Vegetable	Vegetable
Amaranth	-Red Meat-	Trout	Asparagus	-Squash-
Barley	Beef	Tuna-Fresh	Beans	Summer Squ
Buckwheat	Lamb	Tuna-Canned	Beets	Butterbar
Kamut	Pork	Tuna-Oil	Broccoli	Chayote
Millet	Veal	Tuna-Water	BrusselSprouts	Cocozelle
Oats	-Poultry-	-Nuts-	Cabbage	Crooknec
Quinoa	Chicken	Almonds	Carrots	Goldbar
Rye	Cornish Hens	Brazil	Cauliflower	Patty Par
Spelt	Eggs	Cashews	Celery	Yellow
-Rice-	Turkey	Filbet	Chard-Red	Zuchinni
Short Grain	-Fish-	Hazelnut	Chard-White	Winter Squ
Long Grain	Ahi Tuna	Pecan	Collards	Acorn
Jasmine Rice	Bass	Peanuts	Corn	Banana
Basmatic Rice	Catfish	Pine Nuts	Cucumbers	Butternu
Rye	Cod	Walnuts	Dandelions	Cushaw
Spelt	Dover Sole	-Dry Beans-	Endive	Hubbard
-Cold Cereals-	Flounder	Black	Kale	Pumpkin
Amaranth	Haddock	Pinto	-Lettuce-	Spaghett
Kamut Flakes	Halibut	White	Bibb	Turban
Barley Flakes	Mackerel	Lentils	Red Leaf	Sweet Potat
Oats Flakes	Mahi Mahi	Brown	Green	-Tomatoe
Rice-Puffed	Monkfish	Green	Romaine	Yellow Pe
Millet-Puffed	Orange Roughy	Red	Mustard	Red Cher
Almond	Perch	-Split Peas-	Okra	Red Slice
Granola	Petrole Sole	Green	Onions	Lemon Bc
Rye Flakes	Rockfish	Yellow	Parsley	Turnips
-Hot Cereal-	Salmon-Fresh	-Seeds-	Parsnips	Yams
Bits of Barley	Salmon-Canned	Pumpkin	Green Peas	
Barley-Oats-	Sardines	Sesame	Peppers-Bell	
Rice	Sea Bass	Sunflower	Peppers-Hot	
Brown Rice	Shad		Potatoes	
Cream of Rye	Shark		Radishes	
Oat Meal	Smelt		Spinach	
Quinoa Mush	Snapper			
	Sole			
	Swordfish			

0-Circle the items you tried and seem to have no reaction to
X-Cross off the list items you have tried and can not use
S-The items that you had a small reaction to, but okay
?-The items that you are not sure of.

Fruit	Sweetener	Drinks	Snacks	Other
Apricots ○	Amasake ○	-Amazake-	(All Wheat	-Cheese-
Avocado ○	Barley Malt ○	Plain	Free)	Almond/White
Banana	Brown Rice ○	Vanilla	-Brownies-	Almond/Yellow
Blackberries ○	Date Sugar ○	Vanilla Pecan	Carob	Feta-Original
Blueberries ○	Organic Cane ○	-Fruit Juice-	Carob/Raspberry	Goat
Cranberries ○	Fruit Juice ○	Tangerine/Stra	-Cookies-	-Mayonnaise-
Raspberries ○	Granular Fruit	Orange	Double Carob	Canola
Strawberries ○	-Honey-	Guava/Straw	Oatmeal Date	Canola Lite
Cherries ○	Clover	Apple	Sesame Lemon	Eggless
-Citrus-	Alfalfa	Apricot	Butter Almond	Safflower
Grapefruit	Orange	Mango	Ginger Snaps	-Catchup-
Lemons	Other	Pear	Maple Rice	Fruit
Limes	Organic Maple	-Milks-	Lemon Rice	Sweetened
Oranges	Molasses	Almond	-Muffins-	Organic
Tangerines	Sorgum	Oat	Blueberry	Un-Catchup
Tangelos	Stevia	Rice	Carrot	-Oil-
Dates	Dextrose	Soy	Oat	Canola
Figs	Fructose	Sodas	-Snack Bars-	Olive
Grapes	Glucose	Natural	Honey	Safflower
Mangos	Lactose	Lemon Lime	Brazil Nut	Sesame
-Melons-	Maltose	Orange	Macaroon	-Butter-
Cantelope	Mannose	Root Beer	Pine Nut	Canola
Casaba	Corn	Sasparilla	Pumpkin Seed	Safflower
Crenshaw		-Vegetable-	Sesame	Organic Butter
Honeydew		Carrot	-Potato Chips-	Other Butter
Watermelons		Carrot-Beet	Lemon	
Papayas		Carrot-Spina	Pepper	
Peaches		Tomato	Plain	
Pears		TomatoVegie	Rosemary	
Pineapples			-Rice Chips-	
Plums			Plain	
Prunes			Garlic	
Raisins			Herb	
Rhubarb				

Date __01_/_07_/2002__

Dianna's Example

Grains	Meat/Protein	Meat/Protein	Vegetable	Vegetable
Amaranth	*-Red Meat-*	/Trout	Asparagus	*-Squash-*
Barley	Beef	Tuna-Fresh	Beans	*Summer*
Buckwheat	Lamb	Tuna-Canned	Beets	Butterbar
Kamut	Pork	Tuna-Oil	Broccoli	Chayote
Millet	Veal	Tuna-Water	Brussel Sprouts	Cocozelle
S- Oats	*-Poultry-*	*-Nuts-*	Cabbage	Crookneck
Quinoa	Chicken	Almonds	Carrots	Goldbar
Rye	Cornish Hens	Brazil	Cauliflower	Patty Pan
Spelt	Eggs	Cashews	Celery	Yellow
-Rice-	Turkey	Filbet	Chard-Red	Zuchinni
Short Grain	*-Fish-*	Hazelnut	Chard-White	*Winter*
Long Grain	Ahi Tuna	Pecan	Collards	Acorn
Jasmine Rice	Bass	Peanuts	Corn	Banana
Basmatic Rice	Catfish	Pine Nuts	Cucumbers	Butternut
Rye	Cod	Walnuts	Dandelion	Cushaw
Spelt	Dover Sole	*-Dry Beans-*	Greens	Hubbard
-Cold Cereals-	Flounder	Black	Endive	Pumpkin
Amaranth	Haddock	Pinto	Kale	Spaghetti
Kamut Flakes	Halibut	White	*-Lettuce-*	Turban
Barley Flakes	Mackerel	Lentils	Bibb	Sweet Potato
Oats Flakes	Mahi Mahi	Brown	Red Leaf	*-Tomatoes-*
Rice-Puffed	Monkfish	Green	Green	Yellow Pea
Millet-Puffed	Orange Roughy	Red	Romaine	Red Cherry
Almond	Perch	*-Split Peas-*	Mustard	Red Slice
Granola	Petrole Sole	Green	Okra	Lemon Boy
Rye Flakes	Rockfish	Yellow	Onions	Turnips
-Hot Cereal-	Salmon-Fresh	*-Seeds-*	Parsley	Yams
Bits of Barley	Salmon-	Pumpkin	Parsnips	
Barley-Oats-	Canned	Sesame	Green Peas	
Rice	Sardines	Sunflower	Peppers-Bell	
Brown Rice	Sea Bass		Peppers-Hot	
Cream of Rye	Shad		Potatoes	
Oat Meal	Shark		Radishes	
Quinoa Mush	Smelt		Spinach	
	Snapper			
	Sole			
	Swordfish			

0-Circle the items you tried and seem to have no reaction to
X-Cross off the list items you have tried and can not use
S-The items that you had a small reaction to, but okay
?-The items that you are not sure of.

Fruit	Sweetener	Drinks	Snacks	Other
pricots	Amasake	-Amazake-	All Wheat Free	-Cheese-
vocado	Barley Malt	Plain	-Brownies-	Almond/White
anana	Brown Rice	Vanilla	Carob	Almond/Yellow
ckberries	Date Sugar	Vanilla Pecan	Carob/Raspberry	Feta-Original
eberries	Organic Cane	-Fruit Juice-	-Cookies-	Goat
nberries	Fruit Juice	Tangerine/Stra	Double Carob	-Mayonnaise-
pberries	Granular Fruit	Orange	Oatmeal Date	Canola
wberries	-Honey-	Guava/Straw	Sesame Lemon	Canola Lite
herries	Clover	Apple	Butter Almond	Eggless
Citrus-	Alfalfa	Apricot	Ginger Snaps	Safflower
apefruit	Orange	Mango Pear	Maple Rice	-Catchup-
mons	Other	-Milks-	Lemon Rice	Fruit
imes	Organic Maple	Almond	-Muffins-	Sweetened
ranges	Molasses	Oat	Blueberry	Organic
gerines	Sorgum	Rice	Carrot	Un-Catchup
ngelos	Stevia	Soy	Oat	-Oil-
Dates	Dextrose	-Sodas-	-Snack Bars-	Canola
Figs	Fructose	Natural	Honey	Olive
rapes	Glucose	Lemon Lime	Brazil Nut	Safflower
angos	Lactose	Orange	Macaroon	Sesame
Melons-	Maltose	Root Beer	Pine Nut	-Butter-
ntelope	Mannose	Sasparilla	Pumpkin Seed	Canola
asaba	Corn	-Vegetable-	Sesame	Safflower
nshaw		Carrot	-Potato Chips-	Organic Butter
neydew		Carrot-Beet	Lemon	Other Butter
rmelons		Carrot-Spina	Pepper	
payas		Tomato	Plain	
aches		TomatoVegetab	Rosemary	
ears			-Rice Chips-	
eapples			Plain	
lums			Garlic	
runes			Herb	
aisins				
ubarb				

the items that you are not sure of. Do not mark the items that you have not tried. (See "Suggested List Example")

or

Choice B: Copy the items that you like or are not allergic to onto the blank "Suggested List". As you eat the different items, circle the items that you seem to have no problem with, cross off the items that you thought you could use but can't, and put a "S" by the items with a small reaction, and a "?" by the items you are not sure of, but have tried.

Note: Remember our bodies may change over time and even from week to week. What may be acceptable one week may not be the next. Some items you may have to cross off the list forever. Others you can bring back onto the list as a "S" item that you have a small reaction to but is acceptable in limited amounts or over a four-day rotation.

Step 4: Add to the list any item that you may see and try. These items may be grown, purchased, home-made or served at a restaurant. Follow the same marking system as the items that were originally on the list.

Step 5: Revise and check your list each week for the first few months until the items on your list remain almost nearly the same from week to week.

Step 6: After your list is nearly the same for several months, check it only every month or if there is a noticeable change in your health.

My Rotation Diet

Since most items that can be eaten may be eaten in a four-day rotation, the three pages titled "My Rotation Diet", "My Rotation Diet Example #1" and "My Rotation Diet Example #2" are forms to help you plan a four-day rotation of the foods that you can eat.

Directions:

Step 1: Locate the pages which are titled "My Rotation Diet", "My Rotation Diet Example #1" and "My Rotation Diet Example #2".

Step 2: Photocopy the page titled "My Rotation Diet" as needed.

Step 3: Look at the "Suggested List" that you marked in the previous section. Choose one to two different grains and place them in the box under "Day 1" and across from the title "Grain". Choose one to two different grains for "Day 2" and put them in the next box under "Day 2". Choose one to two different grains for "Day 3", and one to two different grains for "Day 4". When you are finished, the top row will be filled grain suggestions. All of the suggestions must be different. If not, choose something else until they are all different. (See "My Rotation Diet Example #1".)

Step 4: Do the same thing for each of the rows titled "Meat/ Protein", "Vegetables Lunch", "Vegetables Dinner", "Fruit', "Sweetener", "Snacks", and "Other". Each of the boxes in a row should be filled with one or two food items that are different from anything else in the rows. (See "My Rotation Diet Example #1".)

Note: In the case of "Meat/Protein", you may be able to do a three day rotation if you choose a different red meat, poultry, and fish for each third day. For example, use chicken the first day. Then, the next time chicken day comes up, use turkey or Cornish game hen instead. The first day fish comes up use catfish. The next time use trout, or another type of fish.

Note: By doing "Meat/Protein" on a three day rotation and the rest of the food items on a four day rotation, you will not have the same vegetables and grain with the same meat/protein each time. It really adds more freedom and variety. (See "My Rotation Diet Example #2")

My Rotation Diet

Date_____/_____/_____

	Day One	Day Two
Grain(s)		
Meat/Protein		
Vegetables Lunch		
Vegetables Dinner		
Fruit		
Sweetener		
Snacks		
Other		
Suspected Food & Reactions		

Day Three	Day Four

Date __01_/_07_/_2002_   Example #1

	Day One	Day Two
Grain(s)	Millet Spelt	Quinoa Potatoes
Meat/Protein	Beef	Chicken
Vegetables Lunch	Asparagus Sweet Potatoes	Brussels Sprouts Chard
Vegetables Dinner	Spinach Carrot Juice	Green Beans Yellow Squash
Fruit	None	None
Sweetener	Other	Honey
Snacks	Lemon Cookies	Macaroon Carrot Muffin
Other	Almond Cheese	Cashew Butter
Suspected Food Reactions	Spelt = Bloating	Honey = "Too Sweet" near end of Macaroon

Day Three	Day Four
Rye Rice	Barley Oats
Fish	Legume
Lettuce Tomatoes	Cauliflower Green Peas
Beet Greens Winter Squash	Broccoli Zucchini
Avocado	None
Rice Malt	Barley Malt
Rice Cookie Rice Bar	Carob Brownie Oatmeal Cookie
Almond Feta Cheese	Pecans Brazil Nuts
Avocado= Roof of mouth itches Rice = Bloated & Gas	Carob ? = Runny Nose Oatmeal = Hard to go down

Date 01 / 07 / 2002   Example #2

	Day One	Day Two
Grain(s)	Millet Spelt	Quinoa Potatoes
Meat/Protein	Beef	Chicken
Vegetables Lunch	Asparagus Sweet Potatoes	Brussels Sprouts Chard
Vegetables Dinner	Spinach Carrot Juice	Green Beans Yellow Squash
Fruit	None	None
Sweetener	Other	Honey
Snacks	Lemon Cookies	Macaroon Carrot Muffin
Other	Almond Cheese	Cashew Butter
Suspected Food Reactions	Spelt = Bloating	Honey = "Too Sweet" near end of Macaroon

Day Three	Day Four
Rye Rice	Barley Oats
Fish	Beef
Lettuce Tomatoes	Cauliflower Green Peas
Beet Greens Winter Squash	Broccoli Zucchini
Avocado	None
Rice Malt	Barley Malt
Rice Cookie Rice Bar	Carob Brownie Oatmeal Cookie
Almond Feta Cheese	Pecans Brazil Nuts
Avocado= Roof of mouth itches Rice = Bloated & Gas	Carob ? = Runny Nose Oatmeal = Hard to go down

Weekly Menu Chart

Most people like to plan at least one week's worth of menus at a time. The "Weekly Menu" and "Weekly Menu Example" will help you plan a week's worth of menus and a list of items to buy.

Directions:

Step 1: Locate the pages which are titled "Weekly Menu" and "Weekly Menu Example".

Step 2: Photocopy the page titled "Weekly Menu" as needed.

Step 3: Looking at the page you filled out titled "My Rotation Diet", select the "Grain" and other food items that you want to eat for breakfast. Place "Day 1" grain in the Sunday "Day 1" Breakfast column. Go down one row and place "Day 1" snack from "My Rotation Diet" to Sunday "Day 1" snack on "Weekly Menu". (See "Weekly Menu Example".)

Note: On the chart, "Breakfast" is followed by "Snack". You can move your snacks to any time of the day you want. Personally, I have two snacks between Lunch and Dinner and rarely snack before Lunch. Some days I even have a snack after Dinner. It really depends on my activities and schedule for the day. Adjust the order of your meals as needed or required.

Step 4: Continue to place items from the "Day 1" column on "My Rotation Diet" list to the Sunday "Day 1" column on the "Weekly Menu" until all of Sunday "Day 1" is complete.

Note: In the real world, one does not usually have time to fix a new "Meat/Protein" each meal. I have found that it is acceptable if you do not have a reaction, to use the leftover "Meat/Protein" from the evening meal the day before for the next day lunch meal. You can also use some properly stored leftovers from several days before.

Note: I have also found ways to fix the lunch vegetables using leftovers too. However, I use vegetable leftovers from a few days ago rather than the day or meal before to keep as large of a time period as possible between eating the same vegetable twice. Also, by not having the same "Vegetable" and "Meat/Protein" together two meals in a row, I find that I have fewer reactions than if I had the exact same meal two times in a row.

Note: If you use leftovers after a couple of days, make sure that they have been stored and handled properly to eliminate any problems with food contamination. Freezing many dishes is a good way to store leftovers.

Step 5: Do the same for Monday, "Day 2" working down the column. Continue with Tuesday, "Day 3", and Wednesday "Day 4" in the same manner. When you get to Thursday, use the "My Rotation Diet" list for "Day 1" again. Friday will use "Day 2", Saturday "Day 3", etc.

Step 6: When you come to Sunday again, continue with the next day in the rotation. So the second Sunday on this plan you would use "Day 4" and Monday would be your next "Day 1". Tuesday "Day 2", Wednesday "Day 3", Thursday "Day 4", Friday "Day 1", and Saturday "Day 2". The third Sunday on this plan would be "Day 3", Monday "Day 4", Tuesday "Day 1", etc.

Note: By doing the rotation this way, you have a variety each Sunday of the month rather than the same meat dish.

Note: If family tradition requires that beef or another item be always served on Sunday or any other day, adjust your rotation to accommodate the tradition. Also, if there is a trip or other occasion that you need to break the rotation, make the necessary adjustments. It is best to keep strictly to this type of rotation, but there are some social situations where one must be flexible. Just remember, the better you are at keeping to the prescribed rotation, the better you will be at eliminating the effects of an allergy reaction.

Step 7: At the bottom of each day, list the items that you will need to buy. When you are selecting quantities of product, remember to plan for leftovers for the next day or two, or for freezing to have future meals prepared in advance.

Weekly Menu Chart

Week of _____ to _____

	Sunday (Day 1)	**Monday** (Day 2)	**Tuesday** (Day 3)
Breakfast			
Snack			
Lunch			
Snack			
Dinner			
To Buy:			

dnesday (Day 4)	Thursday (Day 1)	Friday (Day 2)	Saturday (Day 3)

Week of ___1/06___ to ___1/12___   Example

	Sunday (Day 1)	Monday (Day 2)	Tuesday (Day
Breakfast	Puffed Millet Cereal	Quinoa Waffles	Cooked Rye Cereal
Snack	Lemon Cookie Almond Cheese	Potato Chips	Puffed Rice Square
Lunch	Leftover Fish Asparagus Sweet Potato	Leftover Beef Brussles Sprouts Chard	Leftover Chick Lettuce Tomatoes
Snack	Spelt Bread	Honey Macaroon Cashew Butter	Oatmeal Cool
Dinner	Beef Spinach Carrot Juice	Chicken Green Beans Yellow Squash	Fish Beet Greens Winter Squas
To Buy:	Beef Spinach Almond Cheese	Brussles Sprouts Cashew Butter Quinoa Flour	Lettuce Fish

dnesday (Day 4)	Thursday (Day 1)	Friday (Day 2)	Saturday (Day 3)
Hot Barley Cereal	Millet Waffles	Quinoa Cereal	Puffed Rye Cereal
Sesame Cookie	Lemon Cookie Almond Cheese	Potato Chips	Puffed Rice Square
Leftover Fish Cauliflower Green Peas	Leftover Beef Asparagus Sweet Potato	Leftover Chicken Brussles Sprouts Chard	Leftover Fish Lettuce Tomatoes
arob Brownie	Spelt Bread	Honey Macaroon Cashew Butter	Oatmeal Cookies
Beef Broccoli Zucchini	Chicken Spinach Carrot Juice	Fish Green Beans Yellow Squash	Beef Beet Greens Winter Squash
Broccoli arob Brownies Cauliflower	Carrot Juice Asparagus Sweet Potatoes Chicken	Fish Green Beans Potato Chips	Winter Squash Oatmeal Cookies Puffed Rice Squares

Check-Off Chart

A check-off chart entails no advance planning of menus, but uses only record keeping and a well stocked pantry.

Directions:

Step 1: Locate the pages which are titled "Check-Off Chart", and "Check-Off Chart Example".

Step 2: Photo Copy the page titled "Check-Off Chart". Enlarge if necessary.

Step 3: List down the left column starting with the grains, all of the grains listed on the "suggested list" that you can use. (List alphabetically for ease of locating.) See "Check-Off Chart Example"

Step 4: Then, list your "Meat/Protein"under the grains in alphabetical order.

Step 5: Do the same for vegetables, fruits, sweeteners, drinks, snacks, and other categories.

Step 6: At the end of a meal or at the end of the day, place a check in the column and row representing the food and the calendar day it was eaten. For example, the day of the month is the 11th, the protein is beef, and the vegetables are carrots and green beans. If you want to indicate the meal it was eaten, put "B" for Breakfast, "S" for snack, "L" for Lunch, and "D" for dinner.

Step 7: When you want something to fix for dinner the next day (the 12th), you would look at the chart and decide which protein you have not had for the last two days. In this example, it would be chicken. Then you would look at the vegetables. Any vegetable not checked off in the last two days is available to fix. In this example, chard and zucchini are two choices.

Step 8: Continue through the month in the same manner, looking at and selecting items that you have not eaten in the last two days and then choosing from those items. At the end of the month, start a new chart.

Check-Off Chart

Food

Day
1 2 3 4 5 6 7 8 9 10 11 12 13 14 15 16 17 18 19 20 21 22 23 24 25 26 27 28 29 30 31

Grain

Meat/Protein

Vegetables

Fruits

Snacks/Other

Example

Check-Off Chart

B=Breakfast • L=Lunch • D=Dinner • S=Snack

Food	Day 1	2	3	4	5	6	7	8	9	10	11	12	13	14	15	16	17	18	19	20	21	22	23	24	25	26	27	28	29	30	31
Grain																															
Barley			B					B																							
Millet	B				B																										
Quinoa		B				B																									
Rice				B																											
Rye																															
Spelt			B					B																							
Meat/Protein	B				B																										
Beef																															
Chicken																															
Fish																															
Legume																															
Nuts		S		S		S																									
Vegetables																															
Asaragus	D			L				D																							
Beans	L					L	D																								
Beets		D				L																									
Broccoli							L																								
Brussels Sprouts		L			D																										
Butternut	D			L			L																								
Carrots	L			D			L																								
Cauliflower		D				L		L																							
Endive			L				D																								
Lettuce						D																									
Peas		L				D		L																							
Potatoes						D																									
Spinach			D		L																										
Tomatoes																															
Yams			D																												
Yellow Squash					D			D																							
Zuchinni				D																											
Fruits																															
Apricots	S																														
Avacado						S																									
Cranberries			S				S	S																							
Strawberries					S																										
Dates				S																											
Peaches		S																													
Pears									S																						
Snacks/Other																															
Brownies							S																								
Cheese-Almond	S			S			S																								
Cheese-Feta			S			S		S																							
Cookies-Date		S			S																										
Cookies-Ginger			S																												
Cookies-Lemon	S			S			S																								
Cookies-Oatmeal																															
Cookies-Rice																															
Cookies-Tahini							S																								
Muffin-Carrot																															
Muffin-Oat		S			S																										

NOTES

115

Written Menu *A written menu is sometimes easier than a chart.*

Directions:

Step 1: Locate the pages which are titled "Written Menu", and "Written Menu Example".

Step 2: Photo Copy the pages titled "Written Menu".

Step 3: Fill in dates of the week. (See "Written Menu Example".)

Step 4: Fill in the blanks using the suggestions listed in the parenthesis near each line. (See "Sample Menu Example".)

Menus for the week of _____/_____/_____

Monday

    Breakfast - _____ (Some type of grain)

    Lunch - _____ (Meat and two or more vegetables)

    Snack #1 - _____ (Some type of grain)

    Snack #2 - _____ (nuts, nut butter, fruit)

    Dinner - _____ (Meat and two or more vegetables)

    Snack #3 - _____ (grain,nuts, nut butter,candy bar, ice cream, or fruit)

Tuesday

    Breakfast - _____ (Some type of grain)

    Lunch - _____ (Meat and two or more vegetables)

    Snack #1 - _____ (Some type of grain)

    Snack #2 - _____ (nuts, nut butter, fruit)

    Dinner - _____ (Meat and two or more vegetables)

    Snack #3 - _____ (grain,nuts, nut butter,candy bar, ice cream, or fruit)

Wednesday

    Breakfast - _____ (Some type of grain)

    Lunch - _____ (Meat and two or more vegetables)

    Snack #1 - _____ (Some type of grain)

    Snack #2 - _____ (nuts, nut butter, fruit)

    Dinner - _____ (Meat and two or more vegetables)

    Snack #3 - _____ (grain,nuts, nut butter,candy bar, ice cream, or fruit)

Thursday

Breakfast - _____ (Some type of grain)

Lunch - _____ (Meat and two or more vegetables)

Snack #1 - _____ (Some type of grain)

Snack #2 - _____ (nuts, nut butter, fruit)

Dinner - _____ (Meat and two or more vegetables)

Snack #3 - _____ (grain, nuts, nut butter, candy bar, ice cream, or fruit)

Friday

Breakfast - _____ (Some type of grain)

Lunch - _____ (Meat and two or more vegetables)

Snack #1 - _____ (Some type of grain)

Snack #2 - _____ (nuts, nut butter, fruit)

Dinner - _____ (Meat and two or more vegetables)

Snack #3 - _____ (grain, nuts, nut butter, candy bar, ice cream, or fruit)

Saturday

Breakfast - _____ (Some type of grain)

Lunch - _____ (Meat and two or more vegetables)

Snack #1 - _____ (Some type of grain)

Snack #2 - _____ (nuts, nut butter, fruit)

Dinner - _____ (Meat and two or more vegetables)

Snack #3 - _____ (grain, nuts, nut butter, candy bar, ice cream, or fruit)

Sunday

Breakfast - _____ (Some type of grain)

Lunch - _____ (Meat and two or more vegetables)

Snack #1 - _____ (Some type of grain)

Snack #2 - _____ (nuts, nut butter, fruit)

Dinner - _____ (Meat and two or more vegetables)

Snack #3 - _____ (grain, nuts, nut butter, candy bar, ice cream, or fruit)

Written Menu

Sample Menus for the week of January 12 -16.

Monday

    Breakfast - Millet (hot/cold cereal, or bread)

    Lunch - Leftover fish, tomato, lettuce salad

    Snack #1 - Two slices of spelt bread

    Snack #2 - An organic apple

    Dinner - Roast beef, asparagus, tomato slices

    Snack #3 - Two slices of spelt bread or one pudding, or a serving of nuts

Tuesday

    Breakfast - Quinoa (hot/cold cereal, or bread)

    Lunch - Leftover roast, cold cooked broccoli with a twist of lemon, carrots

    Snack #1 - Cashew butter, 1/3 cup

    Snack #2 - An organic orange

    Dinner - Baked chicken with dill and lemon, yellow squash, green beans

    Snack #3 - French fried potatoes

Wednesday

    Breakfast - Rye (hot/cold cereal, or bread)

    Lunch - Leftover chicken, tomatoes, fresh green pea salad

    Snack #1 - Two slices of rye bread

    Snack #2 - Some organic strawberries

    Dinner - Baked fish, baked winter squash, green leafy vegetable (spinach, chard beet greens)

    Snack #3 - Two slices of rye bread or one pudding, or a serving of fruit

Thursday

    Breakfast - Rice (hot/cold cereal, or bread)

    Lunch - Leftover fish, tomatoes, lettuce, carrot salad

    Snack #1 - One serving of rice chips

    Snack #2 - An organic apple or applesauce (even bake an apple the night before)

    Dinner - Spaghetti with beef (using rice spaghetti), tossed salad, Brussels sprouts

    Snack #3 - Rice-based ice cream

Friday

    Breakfast - Barley (hot/cold cereal, or bread)

    Lunch - Leftover spaghetti

    Snack #1 - Two slices of barley bread

    Snack #2 - A serving of nuts

    Dinner - Chicken stir-fry (chicken, tomatoes, spinach, zucchini)

    Snack #3 - One pudding, or a health bar (Remember all healthy type snacks.)

Saturday

    Breakfast - Oats (hot/cold cereal, or bread)

    Lunch - Leftover chicken stir-fry

    Snack #1 - Two slices of oat bread

    Snack #2 - An organic apple

    Dinner - Baked fish, asparagus, tomato slices

    Snack #3 - Two slices of oat bread or one pudding, or a serving of nuts

Sunday

    Breakfast - Millet (hot/cold cereal, or bread)

    Lunch - Leftover fish, broccoli, tomatoes

    Snack #1 - Two slices of spelt bread

    Snack #2 - A serving of nuts

    Dinner - Roast beef, green leafy vegetable (spinach, chard, beet greens), tomato

    Snack #3 - Two slices of spelt bread or one pudding, or a piece of fruit

Food for Thought...

A recent news item on Paul Harvey News told of a woman in the British Isles who has become allergic to the Twentieth Century and, more specifically, to computer chips.

Experts there had determined that her brain and body were not strong enough to counteract the effects of the electromagnetic frequencies given off by the computer chips and that they were interfering with her body's own electrical system.

As a result, she could not use any modern conveniences that contained a computer chip, including TVs, cars, and phones.

Debate has waged for years on the safety of high power transmission lines, cell phones, microwave ovens, and the safety of computer display screens.

Professional companies even exist who specialize in shielding offices and apartments from too much electromagnetic interference.

Claims of cell phones, high power transmission lines, microwave ovens, and computer terminals causing health problems or cancers have surfaced and some have gone to court. However, most scientific studies claim "no proved connection" to any of these electromagnetic sources and health concerns.

It is interesting to note, however, that the auto-immune diseases chronic fatigue syndrome and fibro-myalgia started appearing shortly after the introduction of the micro-computer to homes and work, approximately 1983. Also, multiple chemical sensitivity and other auto-immune type illness have increased since wide spread computer chip usage.

Among friends and associates who have allergies or other auto-immune health problems, many complain of the same symptoms. Headaches when driving under high power transmission lines, headaches or unexplained weakness after using a cell phone or other wireless devices, fluttering of the chest near microwave ovens in use (without a pacemaker,) weakness or headaches after using computer or computer chip devices, and not being able to wear a quartz-movement wrist watch.

It is interesting to note that these same friends and associates have independently discovered that energy rebalancing exercises such as Tai-Chi and Qi-Gong have been the most helpful treatment.

However, many questions still need to be answered. Are people with allergies and compromised immune systems more sensitive to this type of electromagnetic interference? Or, do these electromagnetic interferences compromise the immune system and allow the body to have more allergies? What connections are there, if any?

Certainly all of the answers are not available and may not be for many years. Some people may be affected and some not. It is a very new question. Our bodies are amazingly complex and we are learning new things everyday about them. But, you are the best judge of how you react to these things. If you get headaches around powerlines, choose a different roadway if possible. If you get dizzy using a cell phone, or a pager, don't use them. If quartz watches bother you, try a wind-up one. When using a computer, if it bothers you, try shielding it (screens are available in computer stores.) And, don't use microwave ovens.

Try Tai-Chi or Qi-Gong exercises. If you feel better, do it. You be the judge. You know your body better than anyone else.

Truly, this field of possible interference with our health is just beginning to be explored. The answers are still out. But, it may just be something worth watching!

Appendix

Plants

In scientific classification at a detailed level, plants can be divided into divisions, sub-divisions, classes, sub-classes, orders, families, sub-families, variants, groups, and tribes. This detailed division can become awkward when trying to keep things simple and easy. So for this book, I will start dividing at the order level.

I have chosen this level of division because I have noted that many times different families of foods I react to are all in the same order.

Order Coniferales
    PINE FAMILY-juniper, pine nuts

Order Ginkoales
    GINKO FAMILY-ginko bilboa

Order Piperales
    PEPPER FAMILY-black pepper, white pepper

Order Proteales
    PROTEA FAMILY-macadamia nut

Order Urticales
    MULBERRY FAMILY-breadfruit, fig, mulberry
    HEMP FAMILY-hops

Order Polygonales
    BUCKWHEAT FAMILY-buckwheat, rhubarb, sorrel

Order Juglandales
    WALNUT FAMILY-black walnut, English walnut, hickory nut, pecan, white walnut (butternut)

Order *Fagales*
  BEECH FAMILY-chestnut
  BIRTCH FAMILY-filbert, natural wintergreen flavor

Order *Chenopodiales*
  GOOSEFOOT FAMILY-beet, chard, quinoa, spinach, sugar beet (beet sugar)
  AMARANTH FAMILY-amaranth

Order *Ranales*
  NUTMEG FAMILY-mace, nutmeg
  LAUREL FAMILY-avocado, bay leaf, cinnamon, sassafras

Order *Papaverales*
  POPPY FAMILY-caper, poppyseed
  MUSTARD FAMILY-arugula, bok choi, broccoli, Brussels sprouts, cabbage, canola, cauliflower, collards, cress (curly, garden, water) horseradish, kale, kohlrabi, mustard (greens, seed), radish (black, Daikon), rutabaga, turnip

Order *Rosales*
  GOOSEBERRY FAMILY-gooseberry, true currant
  ROSE FAMILY-blackberry, boysenberry, dewberry, Loganberry, raspberry, strawberry
  APPLE FAMILY-apple (cider, cider vinegar), loquat, pear, quince, rosehip
  PLUM FAMILY-almond, apricot, cherry, nectarine, peach, plum
  PEA FAMILY-alfalfa, beans [adzuka, asparagus (or yardlong), black, fava, garbanzo, green (or snap), kidney, lima, locust (carob), mung, navy, pinto, soy, wax, white], gums (acacia, arabic, guar, tragacanth), lentil, licorice, peanut, peas [black-eyed (cowpea), chick-pea (garbanzo bean), green (English, snow, sugar)], kudzu, tamarind

Order *Gerinales*
  FLAX FAMILY-flaxseed (and oil)
  SPURGE FAMILY-castor oil, sweet cassava, tapioca
  RUE (CITRUS) FAMILY-citron, clementine, grapefruit, kumquat, lemon, lime, mandarin, orange, pumel lo, tangerine, tangelo, ugli fruit

Order *Salpindales*
  CASHEW FAMILY-cashew, mango, pistachio
  HOLLY FAMILY-yerba mate
  MAPLE FAMILY-maple sugar, syrup

Order Rhamnales
GRAPE FAMILY-grape (and its products: cream of tartar, commercial currants, raisins, wine, wine vinegar)

Order Malvales
MALLOW FAMILY-cottonseed, hibiscus, okra
STERICULA FAMILY-chocolate, cocoa, kola-nut

Order Guttiferales
DILLENIA FAMILY-kiwi fruit

Order Parietales
TEA FAMILY-black, green
PASSION FLOWER FAMILY-passion fruit
PAPAYA FAMILY-papaya

Order Myrtales
MYRTLE FAMILY-allspice, cloves, eucalyptus, guava
EVENING PRIMROSE FAMILY-evening primrose oil
POMEGRANATE FAMILY-pomegranate (also grenadine)
SAPUCAYA FAMILY-Brazil nut

Order Umbellales
GINSENG FAMILY-ginseng
PARSLEY FAMILY-anise, caraway, carrot, celeriac, celery (seed, stalk, and leaf), chervil, cilantro, coriander, cumin, dill, fennel, parsley, parsley root, parsnip

Order Ericales
BLUEBERRY FAMILY-blueberry, cranberry, huckleberry

Order Ebenales
EDONY FAMILY-persimmon
SAPODILLA FAMILY-chicle (chewing gum base)

Order Gentianales
OLIVE FAMILY-black, green, oil

Order Polemoniales
MORNING GLORY FAMILY-jicama, sweet potato, yam
MINT FAMILY-basil, marjoram, mint, oregano, peppermint, rosemary, sage, savory, spearmint, thyme
POTATO FAMILY-eggplant, paprika, pepper (Anaheim, banana, bell, cayenne, cherry, chili, jalapeno), tamarillo, tobacco, tomato, white potato

Order Rubiales
MADDER FAMILY-coffee

Order Curcurbitales
GOURD FAMILY-chayote, cucumber, melons (cantaloupe, casaba, crenshaw, honeydew, muskmelon, Persian melon, water-melon), pumpkin (and seeds), spaghetti squash, summer squashes (crookneck, straightneck, patty pan, yellow, zucchini), winter squashes (acorn, banana, buttercup, butternut, delicata, hubbard)

Order Campanulales
COMPOSITE FAMILY

Group Tubuliflorae
Tribe Helianthene-Jerusalem artichoke, sunflower (oil and seeds)

Tribe Anthemidene-chamomile, stevia, tarragon

Tribe Cynareae-burdock, cardoon, echinacea, globe artichoke, safflower

Group Liguliflorae
Tribe Chichorieae-Belgian endive, chicory, dandelion, endive, escarole, lettuce, salsify

Order Tubiflorate
PEDALIUM FAMILY-sesame (meal, oil, and seeds)

Order Plantasinales
PLANTAGINACEAE FAMILY-psyllium seed

Order Graminales
SEDGE FAMILY-water chestnut

GRAIN FAMILY

Subfamily Poateae
Tribe Bambuseae-bamboo shoots

Tribe Hordeae-barley, kamut, rye, spelt,triticale, wheat

Tribe Aveneae-oats

Tribe Festuceae-lemon grass, teff

Tribe Orizeae-rice, wild rice

Subfamily Panicateae
Tribe Paniceae-millet

Tribe Andropogoneae-milo, molasses, sorghum, sugarcane (cane sugar)

Tribe Tripsaceae-corn, popcorn

Order Palmales
PALM FAMILY-coconut, date, date sugar, sago

Order Arales
ARUM FAMILY-taro

Order Xyridales
PINEAPPLE FAMILY-pineapple

Order Liliales
LILLY FAMILY-aloe vera, asparagus, chives, garlic, leeks onion, sarsaparilla, shallot

YAM FAMILY-true yam

AGAVE FAMILY-agave, yucca

IRIS FAMILY-saffron

Order Scitaminales
BANANA FAMILY-banana, plantain

GINGER FAMILY-cardamon, ginger, tumeric

ARROWROOT FAMILY-arrowroot

Order Orchidales
ORCHARD FAMILY-vanilla

Food Animals

The scientific classification of food animals can involve great detail with phylum, sub-phylum, classes, sub-classes, super-order, order, sub-order, family, and sub-family. To keep things relatively simple, I will start at the order level of classification.

Order Filibranchia
  MUSSEL FAMILY-mussel
  SCALLOP FAMILY-scallop
  OYSTER FAMILY-oyster

Order Eulamellibranchia
  THICK-SHELLED CLAM FAMILY-thick shelled clams
  SOFT-SHELLED CLAM FAMILY-soft shelled clams
  COCKLE FAMILY-cockle

Order Dibranchia
  SQUID FAMILY-squid, cuttlefish

Order Octopoda
  OCTOPUS FAMILY-octopus

Order Decapoda
  PRAWN FAMILY-prawn, shrimp
  LOBSTER FAMILY-crayfish, lobster
  CRAB FAMILY-crab

Order Acipenseroidei
  STURGEON FAMILY-sturgeon (caviar)

Order Isopondyli
  HERRING FAMILY-herring, sardine, shad
  ANCHOVY FAMILY-anchovy
  SALMON FAMILY-salmon, trout
  SMELT FAMILY-smelt
  WHITEFISH FAMILY-whitefish

Order Haplomi
  PIKE FAMILY-blackfish, pickerel, pike

Order Ostariophysi
  SUCKER FAMILY-sucker
  MINNOW FAMILY-carp, chub, minnow
  CATFISH FAMILY-freshwater catfish
  SEA CATFISH FAMILY-sea catfish

Order Acanthini
  CODFISH FAMILY-cod (scrod), haddock, pollack, whiting

Order Berycomorphi
ROUGHY FAMILY-orange roughy
Order Percomorphi
BUTTERFISH FAMILY-butterfish
SEABASS FAMILY-grouper, seabass
DOLPHINFISH FAMILY-Mahi Mahi
PERCH FAMILY-perch, walleye
SNAPPER FAMILY-red snapper
SUNFISH FAMILY-black bass, crappie, freshwater bass, sunfish
MACKEREL FAMILY-mackerel
TUNA FAMILY-albacore, tuna
SWORDFISH FAMILY-swordfish
SAILFISH FAMILY-marlin, sailfish
Order Heterosomata
TURBOT FAMILY-turbot
HALIBUT FAMILY-halibut
FLOUNDER FAMILY-dab, flounder
SOLE FAMILY-sole
Order Salientia
FROG FAMILY-frog
Order Struthioniformes
OSTRICH FAMILY-ostrich
Order Casuariiformes
EMU FAMILY-emu

Order Anseriformes
DUCK FAMILY-duck (and their eggs), goose (and their eggs)
Order Galliformes
GROUSE FAMILY-grouse (partridge)
PHEASANT FAMILY-chicken (and their eggs), Cornish hen, pheasant, quail
TURKEY FAMILY-turkey (and their eggs)
GUINEA FOWL FAMILY-Guinea hen (and their eggs)
Order Columbiformes
DOVE FAMILY-dove, pigeon (squab)
Order Lagomorpha
HARE FAMILY-rabbitt
Order Rodentia
SQUIRREL FAMILY-squirrel
Order Artiodactyla
SWINE FAMILY-pig (pork), wild boar
DEER FAMILY-caribou, deer (venison), elk, moose, reindeer
PRONGHORN FAMILY-pronghorn
ANTELOPE FAMILY-antelope
CATTLE FAMILY-beef (and their milk), bison (American buffalo), ox, goat (and their milk), sheep (and their milk)

References and Suggested Readings

_____(Jan. 25, 2000) "Ban is Proposed on Additive MTBE." Arizona Republic Newspaper, Phoenix, Arizona.

_____ (May 24, 2000) "Water: It Pays to Know What's On Tap." Buyer's Edge-Arizona Republic Newspaper, Phoenix, Arizona.

Associated Press (Feb. 23, 2000) "Gas Additive MTBE May Come Under Toxics Regulation." Arizona Republic Newspaper, Phoenix, Arizona.

Associated Press (April 29, 2000) "Altered Potatoes Don't Cut it as Fast-Food Fries." Arizona Republic Newspaper, Phoenix, Arizona.

Associated Press (Apr.29, 2000) "EPA Approves 1st Ever Biopesticide." Arizona Republic Newspaper, Phoenix, Arizona.

Associated Press (Apr.29, 2000) "Kellogg Wins Anti-Biotech Battle." Arizona Republic Newspaper, Phoenix, Arizona.

Associated Press. (May22, 2000) "State's Cotton is Key in Biotech Dispute." Arizona Republic Newspaper, Phoenix, Arizona.

Associated Press. (June 3,2000) "Common insecticide faces household ban." Arizona Republic Newspaper, Phoenix, Arizona.

Barkie, Karen E. (1982) Sweet and Sugar-Free-An All-Natural Fruit-Sweetened Dessert Cookbook. St. Martin's Press, NY. NY.

Barkie, Karen E. (1985) Fancy, Sweet & Sugar-Free-All-Natural, Fruit-Sweetened Dessert Cookbook. St. Martin's Press, NY. NY.

Brody, Jane E. (Nov, 4, 1999) "Evidence Growing on Relationship Between Diet, ADHD." Arizona Republic Newspaper, Phoenix, Arizona.

Carson, Rachel (1962). Silent Spring. Houghton Mifflin Co. New York

Cartensen, Michelle (August 28, 1998) "Industrial Uses for Crops of the Great Lake Region." http://www.ilsr.org/carbo/ps/factsh14.html

Cheney, Susan Jane (October 1998) "How Sweet it Is." Vegetarian Times

City of Phoenix (1999) "Phoenix Water Services Department 1999 Water Quality Annual Report." City of Phoenix, Az.

de Lange, Jaques Ph.D. (1994). SeaSalt's Hidden Powers-The Biological Action of

All Ocean Minerals on Body and Mind. Happiness Press. Magalia, CA

DuBelle, Lee (1985). Proper Food Combining Phoenix, AZ.

Dumke, Nicolette M. (1997) 5 Years Without Food. The Food Allergy Survival Guide. Adapt Books. Louisville, Colorado.

Dumke, Nicolette M. (1992) Allergy Cooking with Ease-The No Wheat, Milk, Eggs, Corn, Soy, Yeast, Sugar, Grain, and Gluten Cookbook. Starburst Publishers. Lancaster, PA.

Erickson, Jim (May 18, 2000) "Anti-biotech Groups Declare War on Genetically Engineered Cotton." ARN, P.A.

Gannett News Service (May 29, 2000) "Bug Sprays Facing Ban." ARN, P.A.

Grogan, John and Lona Cheryl (February 2000) "The Problem With Genetic Engineering." Organic Gardening

Hermann, William (Mar. 19, 2000) "Chemical Allergies Have Woman Stuck In Tent." Arizona Republic Newspaper, Phoenix, Arizona.

Howard, John (Jan. 23, 2000) "Gas Additive Poses Cruel Choice: Clean Air or Clean Water?" Arizona Republic Newspaper, Phoenix, Arizona.

Jones, Melissa L. (June 7, 1999) "Cure for Camp Verde." Arizona Republic Newspaper, Phoenix, Arizona.

Jones, Melissa L. (June 7, 1999) "Sick Buildings Not Uncommon." Arizona Republic Newspaper, Phoenix, Arizona.

Journal of the American Medical Association (May 5, 1998) "Low-Salt Diet Gets Low Marks." JAMA

Keirsey, David & Bates, Marilyn (1978). Please Understand Me-Character and Temperament Types. Prometheus Nemesis Book Company. Del Mar, CA.

Kroeger, Otto & Janet M. Thuesey (1988). Type Talk - The 16 Personality Types That Determine How We Live, Love, & Work. Delta Book/Dell Publishing/Bantam Doubleday Dell Pub Group N.Y., N.Y.

Lipson, Elaine (June 1998) "Kids overexposed to Pesticides in Food." Delicious!

Magruder, Janie (May 8, 2000) "Living With Allergies to Foods." Arizona Republic Newspaper, Phoenix, Arizona.

Maine, Sandy (4th Printing) (1995) The Soap Book - Simple Herbal Recipes. Interweave Press Inc. Loveland, CO.

Marsden, Kathryn (1999) Food Combining, A Step-by-Step Guide. Elements Book Inc. Boston, MA.

McBarron, M.D., Jan. (Feb/Mar 1999) "Closer Look at Aspartame." Natures Impact

McClary, Heather D.C. D.I.C.C.P. (July/Aug. 1997) Aspartame AKA NutraSweet and Equal. Is This A New Diagnosis to Consider? ICA REVIEW.

McKay, Pat (1992). Reigning Cats and Dogs - Good Nutrition Healthy Happy Animals. Oscar Publications. South Pasadena, California

Meyerowitz, Steve (4th Edition) (1996) Food Combining and Digestion. The Sprout House. Great Barrington, MA.

Morrison, Robert and Boyd, Robert (3rd Edition) (1974) Organic Chemistry. Allyn and Bacon Inc. Boston.

Nebergall, William H. and Schmidt, Frederic C. Et. Al. (3rd Edition) (1968). College Chemistry with Qualitative Analysis. D,C, Heath and Company. Lexington, MA

New York Times (May 6,2000) "Senators Propose End to Gas-Additive Rules." Arizona Republic Newspaper, Phoenix, Arizona.

PepsiCo's (1999) Stockholders Report "Genetically Engineered Foods."

Pitzl, Mary Jo (Mar. 21, 2000) "E.P.A. Pushes Ban on MTBE." Arizona Republic Newspaper. Phoenix, Arizona.

Pitzl, Mary Jo (Apr. 20, 2000) "MTBE Ban Waits for Hulls Signature." Arizona Republic Newspaper. Phoenix, Arizona.

Rapp, Doris J. M.D., F.A.A.A., F.A.A.P. (1991). Is This Your Child? - Discovering and Treating Unrecognized Allergies in Children and Adults William Morrow and Company Inc., NY.

Ridley, Kimberly (Sept/Oct 1998) "A Real Food Revolution>" HOPE

Riotte, Louise (1975) Carrots Love Tomatoes. Garden Way, Pownal, VT

Riotte, Louise (1983) Roses Love Garlic. Garden Way, Charlotte, VT

Roberts, H. J. (1990). Aspartame. Is It Safe? The Charles Press. PA

Ropp, Thomas (May 30, 1999) "Water Dehydration High." Arizona Republic Newspaper. Phoenix, Arizona

Ropp, Thomas (Sept. 20,1999) "Running Tests on Water Filters."Arizona Republic Newspaper. Phoenix, Arizona

Rosenast, Eleanor S. (1993). Soup Alive! Woodbridge Press. Santa Barbara, CA.

Schmitt, Walter H. Jr. (1995). Get These Out of Your Family's Kitchen!

Slivka, Judd (Apr.23,2000) "Years later, D.D.T. still found in the valley fish." Arizona Republic Newspaper. Phoenix, Arizona

Smith, Melissa Diane (Dec. 1997). " Curb Your Carbohydrates Cravings. " Delicious!

Smith, Melissa Diane (Dec. 1997). " The Fats You Need." Delicious!

Turner, Lisa (April 1999) "5 Reasons to Go Organic." Better Nutrition

USA Today (October 28, 1999) "Insecticide Falls Under Scrutiny" Arizona
Republic Newspaper. Phoenix, Arizona

Washington Post (March 17, 2000) "3M Quits Making Stain Repellents." Arizona
Republic Newspaper. Phoenix, Arizona

Walker, Norman W. Dr. (1970). Fresh Vegetable and Fruit Juices - What's miss-
ing in your body? Norwalk Press. Prescott Arizona

Web Reviews (May 7, 2000) Access Magazine Arizona Republic Newspaper.
Phoenix, Arizona www.accessmagazine

Webb, David A (5th Ed) (1988). Making Potpourri, Soaps & Colognes.- 102
Natural Recipes. TAB Books. Blue Ridge Summit, PA.

Webb, David A. (1992). Easy Potpourri. Tab Books. Blue Ridge Summit, PA.

Wegener, Henrik C. (May 20, 1990) "The Consequences for Food Safety of the
Use of Fluoroquinolones in Food Animals," New England Journal of
Medicine-Vol.340 #20 p.1581-2

Wild Oats. "Your Guide to Alternative Sweeteners-Serious Sweet Options" Wild
Oats Inc. 1996

Wild Oats (April 2000) "Do You Want To Know If You're Eating Genetically
Engineered Foods?" www.wildoats.com

Winter, Ruth M.S. (4th Edition) (1978). A Consumer's Dictionary of Food
Additives. Crown Trade Paperbacks. NY.

Yepsen, Roger B. Jr. (Ed.) (1984). The Encyclopedia of Natural Insect and Disease
Control. Rodale Press. Emmaus, PA.

Yozwiak, Steve (Jan. 12, 1997). "Toxic 'Demons'Infiltrate Valley's ground water".
Arizona Republic Newspaper. Phoenix, AZ.